ELDER ABUSE AND NURSING

Carol A. Miller, MSN, RN-BC, has cared for older adults in homes, hospitals, hospice settings, a geropsychiatric program, long-term care facilities, and many community-based programs for more than four decades. Her roles have included nurse practitioner, geriatric care manager, clinical nurse specialist, consultant, administrator, interprofessional team member, and staff nurse. In all these roles and settings, she has provided nursing care for hundreds of older adults who are in abusive or potentially abusive situations. Ms. Miller's interest in elder abuse began in 1978 when she served on the staff of the U.S. House of Representatives, Select Committee on Aging and was involved with organizing hearings and developing legislation to address elder abuse at the federal level. Since then, in addition to her clinical practice, she has participated in research and presented at numerous local, state, and national conferences on various aspects of elder abuse and gerontological nursing.

Ms. Miller has held various faculty positions at the Frances Payne Bolton School of Nursing at Case Western Reserve University and a host of other nursing programs. She is widely published in nursing journals and is the sole author of several nursing texts, including *Fast Facts for Dementia Care* (Springer Publishing Company) and *Nursing for Wellness in Older Adults, 7th Edition*, which won a Book of the Year award from the *American Journal of Nursing* in 2015.

ELDER ABUSE AND NURSING

What Nurses Need to Know and Can Do About It

Carol A. Miller, MSN, RN-BC

SPRINGER PUBLISHING COMPANY
NEW YORK

Springer Publishing Company, LLC
11 West 42nd Street
New York, NY 10036
www.springerpub.com

Acquisitions Editor: Elizabeth Nieginski
Senior Production Editor: Kris Parrish
Composition: Westchester Publishing Services

ISBN: 978-0-8261-3152-2
e-book ISBN: 978-0-8261-3153-9

16 17 18 19 20 / 5 4 3 2 1

The author and the publisher of this Work have made every effort to use sources believed to be reliable to provide information that is accurate and compatible with the standards generally accepted at the time of publication. Because medical science is continually advancing, our knowledge base continues to expand. Therefore, as new information becomes available, changes in procedures become necessary. We recommend that the reader always consult current research and specific institutional policies before performing any clinical procedure. The author and publisher shall not be liable for any special, consequential, or exemplary damages resulting, in whole or in part, from the readers' use of, or reliance on, the information contained in this book. The publisher has no responsibility for the persistence or accuracy of URLs for external or third-party Internet websites referred to in this publication and does not guarantee that any content on such websites is, or will remain, accurate or appropriate.

Library of Congress Cataloging-in-Publication Data
Names: Miller, Carol A., author.
Title: Elder Abuse and Nursing : What Nurses Need to Know and Can Do About It / Carol Miller.
Description: New York, NY : Springer Publishing Company, LLC, [2017] | Includes bibliographical references and index.
Identifiers: LCCN 2016017448| ISBN 9780826131522 (print) | ISBN 9780826131539 (ebook)
Subjects: | MESH: Elder Abuse—prevention & control | Geriatric Nursing—methods | Elder Abuse—diagnosis
Classification: LCC HV6626.3 | NLM WY 152 | DDC 362.6/82—dc23 LC record available at https://lccn.loc.gov/2016017448

Printed in the United States of America by McNaughton & Gunn.

I dedicate this book to the memory of my dear friend and colleague, Betty Lau, whose pioneering work in elder abuse set the wheels in motion for national legislation to address elder abuse. On a clinical level, it was a privilege to work with Betty as one of the many professionals who not only cared about preventing elder abuse, but also took action to address the needs of older adults who were in actual or potential elder abuse situations.

Perhaps most importantly, I dedicate this book to older adults, with the hope that nurses and other professionals will apply the content to prevent elder abuse and address the consequences as we provide care.

CONTENTS

CONTRIBUTORS AND REVIEWERS

CONSULTANT AND REVIEWER FOR THE BOOK

Georgia J. Antezberger, PhD, ACSW

CONTRIBUTORS, CHAPTER 14

BENJAMIN ROSE INSTITUTE ON AGING (BRIA)
Farida Kassim Ejaz, PhD, LISW-S
Christine Foley, BA, RN, COS-C
Lauren Borato, BS
Amanda McLaughlin, BA

CONTRIBUTOR, CHAPTER 13, CASE OF "JANE"

Georgia J. Anetzberger, PhD, ACSW

CONTRIBUTORS, EPILOGUES

Georgia J. Anetzberger, PhD, ACSW
Terry Fulmer, PhD, RN, FAAN

REVIEWER, CHAPTER 5

Charles P. Mouton, MD, MS

REVIEWER, CHAPTER 7

Farida Kassim Ejaz, PhD, LISW-S

FOREWORD

The United States is experiencing a substantial growth in the number of adults age 65 and older and this trend is expected to continue over the next few decades. Although the focus has been on discovering ways to provide the best health care for a population in which the majority will have one or more chronic diseases, little attention has been given to the growing problem of elder abuse. Elder abuse is a worldwide problem with a varying prevalence, based on population settings, definitions, and research studies. Elder abuse is prevalent among older adults with dementia, minority populations, and marginalized populations. However, elder abuse can happen to anyone (e.g., lower or upper socioeconomic status, male or female) and in any setting (e.g., in the home, in long-term care). The National Center on Elder Abuse defines the following seven types of elder abuse: self-neglect, neglect, physical, emotional (psychological), exploitation, sexual, and abandonment.

Elder abuse, also called elder mistreatment or elder maltreatment, is highly associated with death as well as many health problems related to the abuse (e.g., depression, emotional trauma, poor quality of life). In a cost-conscious health care environment, elder abuse can significantly contribute to health care costs with incalculable costs relating to the multifaceted effects on older adults. Health care professionals are uniquely positioned to screen, detect, and intervene for elder abuse; however, a major problem is that many health care professionals lack the knowledge and skills to effectively engage in these activities. In part, this is due to a strong focus on child abuse and domestic violence among younger adults, rather than recognizing the critical issue of elder abuse. Even though these are extremely important issues, elder abuse deserves as much or more attention because of the rapidly growing older population. Up until now, there have been no distinct and comprehensive resources for nurses to guide them on how to identify and intervene in cases of actual or potential elder abuse. Fortunately, Carol A. Miller has integrated current best available evidence and her extensive experience as a gerontological nurse to author *Elder Abuse and Nursing: What Nurses Need to Know and Can Do About It*. This book is a great resource for practicing nurses who play an instrumental role in addressing elder abuse.

This book takes a unique perspective by discussing cultural considerations, key components of physical and psychosocial assessment, and evidence-based interventions across various care settings. In addition, the exemplars presented through the stories of abused older adults will enhance critical thinking skills for easier application to clinical practice. The recognition of elder abuse is important, but just as vital is engaging in preventive measures by identifying vulnerable older adults; preventive strategies are distinctly presented in this book. The book presents the essential role of nurses related to detecting and preventing elder abuse. Elder abuse is under-recognized and underreported, thus limiting nurses' comprehension of the true complexity of the problem. Even though nurses are required by law to report suspected elder abuse, barriers to reporting can present an extremely challenging ethical and moral dilemma. Throughout my nursing career, I have cared for older adults with chronic kidney disease and have witnessed elder abuse, mostly in the forms of neglect and financial abuse. In 2002, although I had been a nephrology nurse for over a decade, I did not truly comprehend my essential role in identifying and intervening in situations of elder abuse until my patient shared his story. As a new nurse practitioner and member of an interprofessional health care team, I was faced with a moral dilemma that many health care professionals face when making decisions to report elder abuse of someone they have known for years.

Mr. Adams (a fictitious name) was a 78-year-old male with multiple chronic health conditions including end-stage renal disease (ESRD) who was undergoing in-center hemodialysis three times a week. The health care team (nephrologist, nurse practitioner, nephrology nurses, and social worker) had cared for Mr. Adams before he was receiving dialysis and knew him to be a strong and vibrant man who continued to work and enjoy spending time with his much younger wife (who was 57 years old), despite having the interference of thrice-weekly dialysis. This all changed after Mr. Adams fell, fractured his right hip, and underwent surgery that required rehabilitation in a skilled nursing facility. His lengthy recovery time and physical functional decline led to loss of his employment. Over time Mr. Adams, experienced further functional decline and appeared to be sad. One day he disclosed that his wife was drinking more and he presented a situation that was consistent with emotional (psychological) abuse. The health care team met with Mr. Adams and he pleaded with them not to report the abuse. Having known him for years, the health care team made the decision to speak to his wife about receiving counseling, which she agreed to do. For a short time, things appeared to improve, but similar to other cases of abuse this did not last. Eventually, Mr. Adams was hospitalized for other health conditions; while he was hospitalized, his wife relocated to another state with all of his assets, leaving him with just the clothes on his back and his monthly Social Security checks. Mr. Adams was devastated and within 3 months he died alone in a long-term care facility instead of in the home he loved and with the wife he adored by his side.

Mr. Adams's story provides an example of the importance of having the knowledge and skills to address actual or potential elder abuse. The health care team felt a moral obligation to Mr. Adams, so they did not report the elder abuse early enough, which led to devastating consequences. Although at the time of the initial identification of elder abuse the health care team thought they were doing the right thing, after reflecting on the situation they have disclosed regrets about the decision and have vowed that this will never happen again.

Unfortunately, it often takes a negative experience for health care professionals to realize the need to be better informed and gain the skills to take action, which was true in the previous example. Therefore, it is crucial to have a book like this to help nurses recognize elder abuse and implement appropriate interventions that can lead to the best possible outcomes. This book discusses elder abuse within the complexities of different care settings and under unique circumstances. I am extremely grateful for this book because it provides a comprehensive guide of how to address the emerging critical issue of elder abuse.

Debra Hain, PhD, ANP-BC, GNP-BC, FAANP
Associate Professor/Lead AGNP Faculty
Nurse Practitioner, Louis and Anne Green Memory
and Wellness Center
Christine E. Lynn College of Nursing, Florida Atlantic University
Boca Raton, Florida

PREFACE

For more than four decades as a nurse and nurse practitioner, I have cared for older adults in homes, hospitals, hospice settings, a geropsychiatric program, long-term care facilities, and a variety of community-based programs. In all these settings, I have been an integral part of the lives of older adults who experienced some abuse in one or more of its many forms. Sometimes I did not recognize the abuse; sometimes I was powerless to change the situation; sometimes I reported the situation; sometimes the outcomes were not pleasant; and sometimes I was able to resolve the situation. At all times, I knew that I could at least listen to these older adults and support them, no matter how frustrated I was by the many barriers to resolving the abuse or alleviating the consequences. These situations—and the challenges inherent in them—made me keenly aware of the tremendous need for more knowledge, more services, more interventions, and more efforts toward prevention of elder abuse.

In contrast to the commonly held perception that elder abuse occurs primarily in substandard nursing homes or in high-risk domestic situations, the reality is that any older adult can become a victim of elder abuse. Studies indicate that at least 1 of every 10 older adults experiences elder abuse. Most importantly, this statistic does not account for the many other older adults who are at risk for abuse, nor does it include the larger percentage of cases that are unrecognized and unreported. Applying these statistics to health care settings, if you are a nurse who provides care to older adults, you are likely to encounter an elder abuse situation at least occasionally and probably more frequently than you realize. On a personal level, you may know an older friend, neighbor, or family member who is experiencing or has experienced elder abuse.

Elder abuse remains hidden until one of the following scenarios occurs: (a) The situation escalates to a level that requires the attention of professionals who cannot ignore its seriousness; (b) the older adult trusts a caring professional enough to share his or her story and the professional takes action to address the situation; or (c) a caring professional recognizes indicators of abuse and takes appropriate actions. A major intent of this book is to enable nurses to be the caring professionals who recognize indicators of or risks for elder abuse and intervene to prevent or address this all-too-common and very serious health problem.

Throughout this book, stories of older adults illustrate what it means to be a victim of or at risk for elder abuse. The book also describes nurses who care for older adults who are victims of elder abuse. For the most part, the accounts involve "ordinary" older adults and nurses and they represent commonly encountered nurse–client or nurse–patient situations. The nurses are not certified as "elder abuse nurses"—there is no such certification—but they are "everyday nurses" who care for older adults in all health care settings. Sometimes the nurses do not recognize the abuse or the risk of abuse, sometimes they do not know what questions to ask, sometimes they do not want to know the details, sometimes they report the abuse, other times they decide not to report, or they do not even realize that they are obligated to make a report. In some situations, the nurses feel powerless and occasionally they may even be intimidated by the perpetrators, who may also be the caregivers for the older adult. At times, nurses experience moral distress or ethical dilemmas, for example, when they are required to respect a legally competent older adult's right to make unwise decisions that pose risks to health and safety. In these situations, they know what interventions can reduce the risks, but they are not the ones making choices.

I developed this book as a guide for nurses who care for older adults in any clinical setting, with the recognition that they encounter situations of actual or potential elder abuse among their usual clients and patients. These situations are complex and challenging and nurses have no "how-to" manual to guide their care. This book merges my extensive professional background in gerontological nursing with my long-time commitment to preventing and addressing elder abuse. While I recognize that elder abuse requires that solutions be initiated at many levels, I also recognize the essential roles of nurses in addressing elder abuse when they care for older adults. In many situations, nurses are the linchpins of the care plan. My approach in this book is to apply what is known about elder abuse to the everyday experiences of practicing nurses. As such, it is a research-based and clinically relevant guide to what nurses need to know and can do about elder abuse.

OVERVIEW OF THE BOOK

The chapters in Part I provide background information on elder abuse as it applies to nurses in health care settings. Chapter 1 introduces the topic by describing the forms, risks, and consequences of elder abuse in various settings. Issues related to terminology are also discussed, as there is much confusion about terms. Chapter 2 discusses elder abuse by a trusted other in domestic settings. Nurses encounter this type of elder abuse when they care for older adults who live with or receive care from trusted others who neglect, abuse, or exploit them in some way. Chapter 3 describes self-neglect as a unique form of elder abuse and discusses the roles of nurses in addressing these situations. Chapter 4 provides an overview of elder abuse in long-term care facilities and it reviews responsibilities of nurses with regard to this type of abuse. Chapter 5 helps nurses develop cultural competence when caring for older adults who may be in abusive situations. This chapter also provides details about cultural considerations related to elder abuse in specific groups in the United States.

Part II describes roles of nurses in detecting and reporting elder abuse. Chapter 6 discusses legal responsibilities of nurses, including information about reporting suspected abuse. Chapter 7 helps nurses recognize indicators of elder abuse and communicate with older adults and caregivers about this complex and sensitive issue. Chapter 8 focuses on ethical issues related to elder abuse, with emphasis on dilemmas faced by nurses in clinical settings. An additional intent is to discuss self-care for nurses so they become comfortable with their professional responsibilities and personal responses when they care for older adults in abusive situations.

The chapters in Part III serve as a "how-to" guide for nurses. As such, these chapters illustrate the application of usual nursing assessment and intervention skills to unusual situations when nurses care for older adults who are in abusive or potentially abusive situations. Chapter 9 helps nurses apply assessment skills to elder abuse situations, including the following aspects: overall assessment approach, physical assessment, safety and functioning, psychosocial assessment, and caregivers and social supports. Nurses can use information in Chapter 10 to develop nursing interventions that address the following facets of elder abuse situations: overall approach, behavioral and mental health issues, risks to safety of the older adult and others, resources within the health care settings, needs of caregivers, family dynamics, and legal issues. Chapter 11 provides comprehensive information and case examples about resources that nurses can use to address elder abuse.

The chapters in Part IV use unfolding case examples to describe nurses in action addressing elder abuse across settings. Chapter 12 illustrates roles of several nurses as they work with other professionals to address a complex domestic elder abuse situation. Chapter 13 demonstrates the multidimensional roles of Nurse Anne as she provides one-on-one care and as she participates in a multidisciplinary team discussion to address complex issues related to a self-neglecting older adult. Chapter 14 illustrates how Nurse Cathy works with members of an interprofessional team to identify risks and implement interventions to prevent elder abuse.

Part V provides an overview of financial abuse and sexual abuse as types that often involve specialized professionals and law enforcement officers. Chapter 15 provides an overview of financial abuse and describes roles of nurses in identifying and preventing this type of elder abuse. It also presents information about the important roles of health care professionals in identifying the need for a comprehensive financial capacity assessment and facilitating referrals when the need is identified. Chapter 16 discusses aspects of sexual abuse of older adults that are pertinent to nurses, including unique skills related to nursing assessment of and interventions for sexually abused older adults.

Georgia J. Anetzberger, PhD, ACSW, a nationally recognized elder abuse scholar and advocate, developed the first of the two epilogues in the book to present a vision for the future. Her hopeful perspective is rooted in 42 years of work in the field of elder abuse, including her current involvement with numerous ongoing initiatives, such as the Advisory Board for the National Center on Elder Abuse, the Steering Committee of the Elder Justice Roadmap, and the Board of Directors for the National Committee for the Prevention of Elder Abuse. Dr. Anetzberger's epilogue concludes with a call for nurses to take action—now!—to address elder abuse.

Terry Fulmer, PhD, RN, FAAN, contributed an epilogue based on her extensive expertise and leadership in clinical, research, and policy-making roles related to elder abuse. Dr. Fulmer is nationally and internationally recognized as a leading expert in geriatrics and is best known for her research on elder abuse and neglect, which has been funded by the National Institute on Aging and the National Institute for Nursing Research. She recaps major themes of this book and eloquently highlights the responsibilities of nurses in addressing elder mistreatment during "every touch point with our patients, our clients, our residents."

FEATURES OF THIS BOOK

- Guides to nursing assessment and interventions that address specific forms of elder abuse
- Several types of case examples illustrating nurses in action addressing situations of elder abuse across health care settings
- Details about responsibilities of nurses in various health care settings
- Words of older adults describing their experiences and perceptions of elder abuse
- Words and thoughts of nurses describing their reflections on and perceptions of elder abuse situations
- Key Points: What Nurses Need to Know and Can Do

WALKING IN THE SHOES OF NURSES CARING FOR OLDER ADULTS

On a personal/professional note: I have walked in the shoes of nurses who have encountered elder abuse situations and experienced the frustrations of caring for older adults who are at risk for or exhibit the serious consequences of elder abuse, neglect, or self-neglect. From this perspective, I understand the frustrations of being able to anticipate predictable consequences of actions taken or not taken that foster these situations, but being helpless to prevent the consequences. With great sadness, I recall my visit to an older couple who were socially and culturally isolated and overwhelmed with the burden of mutual caregiving due to their progressively declining health problems. I had reported them to adult protective services, but professional actions were too little and too late, and I was troubled when I watched the evening news report that the husband had beaten his wife with a tire iron. Although this experience occurred 30 years ago, I still have vivid memories of my visit to them and the evening news report several days later—and I still have questions about what could have been done to prevent this devastating outcome. I would like to believe that this and other types of elder abuse no longer occur, but I know too well that much progress needs to be made in preventing elder abuse. On a hopeful note, however, I am optimistic about the many efforts of direct-care professionals, administrators, scholars, policy makers, and funding initiatives that are currently underway. My overriding hope is that information in this book will empower nurses to make a major difference in the lives of older adults who are in actual or potential elder abuse situations. Echoing the calls to action articulated by Georgia Anetzberger and Terry Fulmer in the epilogues, I call on nurses to become knowledgeable about elder abuse so they can competently and comfortably apply their nursing skills to caring for older adults who all too commonly are at risk for or experiencing elder abuse.

Carol A. Miller

Carol A. Miller

ACKNOWLEDGMENTS

On a personal level, I am most grateful for the boundless support of my main cheerleader, Pat Rehm, whose mantra for me has been "keep writing." The support and encouragement from my family has been invaluable as I have developed this book. On a professional level, I am especially grateful for the support, guidance, and wisdom provided by Georgia J. Anetzberger and Elizabeth Nieginski from inception to completion of the book. I greatly appreciate Georgia's multidimensional expert consultation and contributions and Elizabeth's ongoing expertise and advice as my editor at Springer Publishing Company. Just as it takes a team to address elder abuse, it takes a team to develop a book, and I appreciate all who have contributed to this process.

I

THE NURSE'S GUIDE TO ELDER ABUSE IN ITS MANY FORMS AND GUISES

INTRODUCTION TO ELDER ABUSE AND NURSING: FORMS, SETTINGS, RISKS, AND CONSEQUENCES

Professional recognition of mistreatment of older adults began during the mid-1970s when physicians in the United Kingdom wrote about "granny battering" as a phenomenon that was similar to "baby battering." Emphasis was on the need to bring this issue to the attention of general practitioners, community nurses, health visitors, and social workers (Baker, 1975; Burston, 1975). Simultaneously in the United States, the noted geriatrician Robert Butler was bringing attention to the "battered old person syndrome," with emphasis on medical aspects of neglect, self-neglect, and physical abuse of older people. Butler drew further attention to elder abuse as an aspect of ageism in his Pulitzer Prize-winning book *Why Survive? Being Old in America* (Butler, 1975). Spurred by this attention to the problem, gerontologists, legislators, social service providers, and health care professionals became interested in this topic, and by the 1990s *elder abuse* was widely recognized as a complex and serious problem that affected many older adults. The 2015 White House Conference on Aging identified elder abuse and neglect as a priority topic with emphasis on the urgent need to address this widespread and serious public health problem and its devastating consequences.

Elder abuse scholars emphasize the urgent need for evidence-informed guidelines related to prevention of and interventions for elder abuse. However, because this aspect of research is still evolving, nurses in clinical practice today have little guidance when they care for older adults who are in situations of actual or potential elder abuse. Guidelines for health care practitioners tend to focus on indicators of physical abuse (e.g., bruises, malnutrition, pressure ulcers) or on legal requirements for reporting suspected cases. Nurses in clinical practice, however, recognize that caring for abused or neglected older adults is much broader and more challenging than identifying indicators and making obligatory reports. Information in this book is based on the best available evidence, with the intent of providing practical ways in which nurses can address broad aspects of elder abuse as a serious and often hidden health issue that affects many older adults for whom they provide care. This chapter discusses the first step, which involves recognizing that elder abuse presents in many guises, occurs in all settings, is caused by numerous interacting variables, and is associated with serious consequences.

FORMS AND DEFINITIONS OF ELDER ABUSE

Elder abuse is important to health care professionals because, at its core, it is "a violation of older adults' fundamental rights to be safe and free from violence and contradicts efforts toward improved well-being and quality of life in healthy aging" (Institute of Medicine and National Research Council, 2014, p. 1). The World Health Organization (WHO, n.d.) defines *elder abuse* as a single or repeated act or lack of appropriate action that (a) occurs within any relationship in which there is an expectation of trust or dependence, and (b) causes harm or distress to an older person. In the United States, elder abuse is defined by state laws, which vary significantly, as discussed in Chapter 6. Specific actions delineated in state laws as representing abuse include neglect, self-neglect, abandonment, exploitation, sexual abuse, undue influence, unreasonable confinement, violation of rights, and denying privacy or visitors. In the United States, the National Center on Elder Abuse (n.d.) defines seven types of elder abuse as follows:

- Self-neglect: behavior of an elderly person that threatens his or her own health or safety, such as failure to provide adequate food and nutrition for oneself or failure to take essential medications
- Neglect: refusal or failure by those responsible to provide food, shelter, health care, or protection for a vulnerable elder
- Physical abuse: inflicting, or threatening to inflict, physical pain or injury on a vulnerable elder, or depriving that individual of a basic need

- Emotional (psychological) abuse: inflicting mental pain, anguish, or distress on an elder person through verbal or nonverbal acts

- Exploitation: illegal taking, misuse, or concealment of funds, property, or assets of a vulnerable elder

- Sexual abuse: nonconsensual sexual contact of any kind, or coercing an elder to witness sexual behaviors

- Abandonment: the desertion of a vulnerable elder by anyone who has assumed responsibility for care or custody of that person

Although this typology is useful for defining seven forms of abuse, it does not describe the complexity of elder abuse as it occurs in different settings and under unique circumstances. Each elder abuse situation involves an older adult who is the victim and a perpetrator who is responsible for the action or inaction leading to neglect or abuse. In situations of self-neglect, the older adult is viewed as both the perpetrator and the so-called victim. When self-neglect occurs, the primary issues usually revolve around safety, health, individual rights, and decision-making abilities of the person who is self-neglecting. Elder abuse involving one or more perpetrator(s) includes a wide spectrum of situations, ranging from unintended neglect due to the inadequacy of caregivers to criminal sexual abuse. When elder abuse situations evolve slowly—which is often the case—it can be difficult to pinpoint an exact time at which a report should be made. Another complicating factor is that legal and ethical issues are often inherent in elder abuse situations, as discussed in Chapter 8.

Definitions of elder abuse are based on research about types, risk factors, victims, perpetrators, relationships between victims and perpetrators, and factors associated with the environments in which elder abuse occurs. Table 1.1 summarizes changes in terminology that evolved based on different research foci between 1975 and 2003. In 1991, Margaret Hudson, a nurse researcher, developed a five-level taxonomy of violence against elders based on the "collective wisdom" of 63 elder mistreatment experts (Hudson, 1991). The experts unanimously endorsed the following conclusions in this landmark study:

- An essential characteristic of any form of elder mistreatment is that it causes physical, psychological, social, or financial harm to the older adult.

- Aging increases a person's vulnerability both to mistreatment and to its harmful effects.

- Ageism, with its implied devaluing of the elderly, increases an older adult's risk of mistreatment.

- Elder mistreatment, abuse, and neglect are relational concepts that must be considered according to the context in which they occur.

Hudson's study and the resulting taxonomy established a foundation for elder abuse scholars to begin addressing many questions related to definitions of elder abuse. Based on an extensive review of studies, Anetzberger (2012) proposed an updated taxonomy addressing elder abuse on the following levels: setting, form, perpetrator motivation, and locus of harm. In Figure 1.1, these concepts are applied in a flow chart to describe the complexity of elder abuse as nurses would address it in clinical settings. Theoretically, all forms of elder abuse can occur in any setting; however, the figure focuses on the scenarios that nurses are most likely to encounter in clinical settings.

From a clinical perspective, it is important to recognize that several types of elder abuse often occur together. For example, an older female adult experiences both physical and emotional abuse when a caregiver grabs her arms and shakes her while threatening to leave her without

TABLE 1.1 Terminology Related to Elder Abuse, 1975 to 2003

TERMINOLOGY	TIME FRAME	FOCUS OF STUDIES
Granny battering	1975–1977	Physical abuse experienced by women
Elder abuse		
Elder mistreatment	1979–1982	Risk factors
Battered elder syndrome		Broader range of actions
Granny battering		
Old age abuse	1984	Widening of victims
Elder mistreatment	1998	Broader range of perpetrators
Elder abuse	2002–2003	Widening of context
Elder mistreatment		

Adapted from Mysyuk, Westendorp, and Lindenberg (2013).

FIGURE 1.1 Framework for understanding elder abuse.

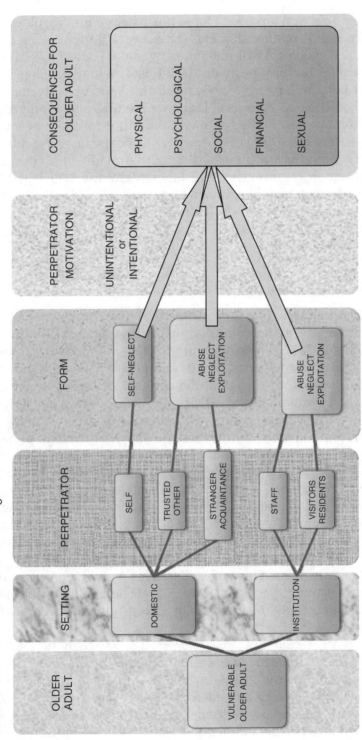

Adapted from Anetzberger (2012).

care if she does not stop asking for so much help. Also, two older adults in a dependent relationship can experience "mutual elder abuse," which often evolves slowly and unintentionally. For example, a spouse who cares for her physically disabled husband may develop dementia; they both become neglected and the husband verbally abuses his wife when she no longer is able to prepare their meals and care for him. A joint project of the National Committee for the Prevention of Elder Abuse and the U. S. Department of Justice is currently addressing *polyvictimization in later life* with the goal of providing training materials on this topic beginning in 2017. Emotional abuse, which perhaps is the most difficult to define, is viewed as underpinning all other forms of abuse, almost as its essence (Taylor, Killick, O'Brien, Begley, & Carter-Anand, 2014).

ISSUES RELATED TO TERMINOLOGY

Elder abuse terminology is problematic in many ways because it has become "a catch-all term for various wrongs against older people" (Anetzberger, 2012, p. 12). In addition, the term *elder abuse* is viewed as ageist and narrowly associated with physical abuse alone, rather than being associated with multidimensional aspects of harm to older adults. From a multicultural perspective, because an "elder" is held in special esteem by many groups, it is disrespectful to combine this term with "abuse." Thus, some researchers and practitioners prefer the phrase *mistreatment of older adults* (Lithwick, Beaulieu, Gravel, & Straka, 2000). Another rationale for preferring terms such as *elder mistreatment* and *elder maltreatment* is to differentiate between types that involve a perpetrator and self-neglect. Self-neglect is considered a separate phenomenon in some laws and in many other countries, but the National Center on Elder Abuse defines it as a type of elder abuse. In this book, the term *elder abuse* is used as the umbrella term inclusive of the seven types currently defined by the National Center on Elder Abuse. As discussed in Chapter 6, state laws vary widely in definitions of elder abuse, and there is currently no universally agreed-upon definition of types of elder abuse.

The terms *victim* and *perpetrator* are also problematic, especially with regard to domestic abuse situations that typically occur in the context of complex and long-term relationships involving love, attachment, resilience, agency, and interdependence (Daniel & Bowes, 2011). These terms evolved as an extension of terminology related to child abuse and interpersonal violence. In laws, policies, and professional literature related to elder abuse, a perpetrator includes people who seriously physically or sexually abuse older adults as well as people who are well-intentioned caregivers with significant personal needs or limitations. In some situations, it is difficult to distinguish between a perpetrator and a victim; for example, when both spouses are impaired and attempt to provide care for each other without necessary supports. As the field of elder abuse research matures, terminology may emerge that is not based on child abuse or interpersonal violence research, but in the interim these terms are widely used—although with some reluctance—in current elder abuse literature and in this book.

Additional issues are associated with the interchangeable and overlapping use of terms for specific types. For example, *emotional abuse* and *psychological abuse* are applied interchangeably to the same type of abuse. Professional references tend to favor the term *psychological abuse* and references for the general public usually refer to *emotional abuse*. When elder abuse occurs in the context of a current or former spousal or committed partnership, it is a form of *domestic violence* and is more specifically called *intimate partner violence* or simply *partner violence.* In some cases of sexual abuse, *rape* is the accurate term. Discussions of *financial abuse* use the term *exploitation* interchangeably, usually in reference to tangible assets or financial resources of the older adult. However, in some state laws, the definition of exploitation includes actions such as coercion of an older adult to perform work against his or her will.

Another consideration related to terminology is that elder abuse definitions vary not only according to state laws within the United States but also internationally. For example, because the WHO (n.d.) defines *elder abuse* within the context of a trust relationship, self-neglect is not considered elder abuse in many countries (e.g., Europe, Australia). The definition of the WHO does not address victimization by strangers or acquaintances. Similarly, self-neglect is not delineated in all state laws on elder abuse, but it may be addressed in adult protective service laws. In this book, self-neglect is discussed in Chapter 3 as domestic elder abuse without a perpetrator and in Chapter 13 as a case example.

PERSPECTIVES OF OLDER ADULTS

Definitions and typologies of elder abuse cited by scholars and organizations may differ from the ways in which older adults themselves perceive and define elder abuse. A systematic review of 15 studies published between 1996 and 2008 emphasized that older adults view elder abuse on both a personal level and a societal level and associate this concept with ageism, disempowerment, and family breakdown (Killick, Taylor, Begley, Carter-Anand, & O'Brien, 2015). Studies based on interviews with community-dwelling older adults provide insight into ways in which older adults conceptualize elder abuse. Several studies point toward emotional abuse as a type that is most commonly experienced and associated with serious consequences but at the same time is a type that is very difficult for researchers or practitioners to address. For example, data from eight focus groups including 58 older adults indicated that "emotional abusiveness was viewed as underpinning all forms of abuse, and as influencing its experienced severity" (Taylor et al., 2014, p. 223). Another study by Naughton, Drennan, and Lafferty (2014) analyzed data from face-to-face interviews with 2,021 older adults and found that slightly more than one fourth of the participants had experienced emotional abuse and described examples as overt behaviors (e.g., threats, demands, bullying, deception) and covert behaviors (e.g., being ignored, undermined, made to feel like a nuisance).

The thing that amazes me about ageism is the way that we treat people who have survived long enough to get old . . . like they're a different species or a different plant and that younger people are not going to get old themselves. (Bowes, Ghizala, & Macintosh, 2012, p. 264)

The bottom line to ageism is that it allows people to be depersonalized and once you're depersonalized . . . then you are all vulnerable to abuse. (Walsh, Olson, Ploeg, Lohfeld, & Macmillan, 2011, p. 27)

Specific issues identified by older adults but rarely addressed in professional references include lack of privacy, loss of independence, denial of rights, being treated like a child, lack of control over own affairs, not being allowed or encouraged to do things for themselves, and being forced to do things against their will (e.g., being "put" in a nursing home). These examples can be categorized as *violations of rights*. In this book, direct quotes from older adults are cited in a feature called "In the Words of an Older Adult" to provide a glimpse of older adults' perceptions of elder abuse.

ESTIMATES OF ELDER ABUSE IN THE UNITED STATES

Because elder abuse is both hidden and multifaceted, reports of incidence or prevalence vary significantly, with recent studies tending to focus on the occurrence of particular types of elder abuse during a specific period of months or years. For example, a nationally representative sample of 5,777 older adults in the United States reported that 1 in 10 community-dwelling Americans who were not cognitively impaired experienced neglect or emotional, physical, or sexual mistreatment during the previous year, with many experiencing it in multiple forms (Acierno, Hernandez-Tejada, Muzzy, & Steve, 2010). In addition, the study found that 5.2% of these older adults reported current financial exploitation by family and 6.5% reported lifetime financial exploitation by a stranger after age 60. Studies that included cognitively impaired older adults reported significantly higher prevalence rates for elder abuse. A recent review of 28 studies of elder abuse toward older adults with dementia found the following prevalence rates: 27.9% to 62.3% for psychological abuse, 3.5% to 23.1% for physical abuse, 20.2% for neglect by caregivers, 15% for financial exploitation, and 13.6% to 18.8% for self-neglect (Dong, Chen, & Simon, 2014). This research review also found that 31% of abused community-dwelling older adults with dementia experienced multiple forms of abuse, 35% of caregivers experienced mutual verbal abuse, and 6% experienced mutual physical abuse.

Researchers and policy makers consistently emphasize that prevalence rates for elder abuse are significantly underestimated because the majority of cases go undetected and unreported. This tip-of-the-iceberg theme has been discussed for decades and was recently substantiated by a report called *Under the Radar: New York State Elder Abuse Prevalence Study*. This large representative study found that for every case of elder abuse that was known to authorities, 23.5 cases were unknown, with financial exploitation having the highest percentage of unreported cases (Lifespan of Greater Rochester, Inc., Weill Cornell Medical Center of Cornell University, & New York City Department for the Aging, 2011).

THE "WHO" AND "WHY" OF ELDER ABUSE

Three of the most complex questions about elder abuse are as follows:

- Which older adults become victims of elder abuse?
- Who are the perpetrators of elder abuse?
- Why does elder abuse happen?

Answers to these questions involve many interacting variables associated with each unique elder abuse situation. Social scientists have long acknowledged that more than three variables interacting with one another in any given situation make that situation extraordinarily complicated and difficult to explain. This theme is echoed in the perspective of elder abuse scholars who view elder abuse as a multifaceted social problem similar to poverty or juvenile delinquency (Anetzberger, 2013). In addition to the inherent complexity of elder abuse situations, research on causation is complicated by the following considerations:

- There is no common definition of elder abuse.
- Causation varies significantly according to the form of abuse.
- Causation varies significantly according to the relational context for self-neglect and abuse by a trusted other.
- Many, if not most, elder abuse situations are unreported and invisible to service providers or researchers.
- Abused older adults rarely are in a position to be included in studies.
- Perpetrators rarely are reliable sources of information.

Harbison and colleagues suggest that the most effective approach to elder abuse as a social problem is to disband the search for an overall unifying theory, "and focus instead on understanding and addressing the range of problems that it represents. In so doing, it will be possible to address a variety of injustices perpetrated against older people and to fully acknowledge the diversity of older generations' needs and capacities" (Harbison et al., 2012, p. 100). This approach is consistent with Anetzberger's recommendation that causation of elder abuse can be addressed by investigating risk factors that are associated with the following: (a) older adults, (b) perpetrators, (c) the relationship between the victim and the perpetrator, and (d) the social environment in which elder abuse takes place. Within this context, she defines *risk factors* as "commonly accepted conditions found through research to be closely linked to the occurrence of elder abuse" (Anetzberger, 2013). Box 1.1 summarizes risk factors for elder abuse that are most often identified in research.

Throughout this book, risk factors for older adults, perpetrators, and the relationships between victims and perpetrators are discussed in the context of types of abuse that nurses commonly address in clinical settings. Specifically, Chapter 2 discusses risk factors for elder abuse in community-based (i.e., domestic) settings, including attention to caregiver stress in relation to causation of elder abuse. Chapter 3 reviews characteristics of older adults at risk for self-neglect, and

BOX 1.1 Risk Factors for Elder Abuse

Risk Factors for Victims and Perpetrators

- Victim: physical dependence, dementia, problem behaviors
- Perpetrator: mental illness (e.g., history of psychiatric hospitalization), alcoholism, hostility in general or directed toward victim, financial or housing dependency
- Relationship between victim and perpetrator: shared living arrangements, social isolation

Risks Factors for Forms of Abuse

- Emotional: low social support, physical dependence, prior traumatic experiences
- Physical: substance abuse, mental illness, social isolation, and unemployment of perpetrator; low social support for victim
- Neglect: low income, poor health, inadequate social support
- Financial: physical disability
- Sexual: low social support, prior traumatic events

Risk Factors for Abuse in Care Facilities

- Facility conditions that increase risk for abuse: no abuse prevention policies, inadequate staff training and screening, high staff turnover, history of complaints
- Facility conditions that increase risk for physical abuse: resident overcrowding
- Resident risk factors: unmet needs, no visitors, physical dependency, cognitive impairment

Adapted from Anetzberger (2013).

Chapter 4 discusses factors that contribute to elder abuse in long-term care settings. Roles of nurses in identifying risk factors in clinical settings are discussed in Chapter 7. Pertinent theories about causation are discussed throughout this book in relation to specific types of elder abuse. The following sections address societal level risk factors and other conditions that most often contribute to the development of elder abuse situations.

SOCIETAL LEVEL RISK FACTORS

The term *ageism* was coined by Robert Butler in 1968 and published the next year (Butler, 1969) to describe prejudices and stereotypes that are applied to older people sheerly on the basis of their age. For several decades, ageism has consistently been identified as a societal level condition that contributes not only to the occurrence of elder abuse but also to the lack of funding for research and services related to all aspects of elder abuse. Older adults themselves identify loss of respect in society that filters down to a personal level as a basis of elder abuse (Taylor et al., 2014). Prejudice and stereotyping of people with disabilities is another societal level factor that is associated with elder abuse. For example, stereotypes about older adults and adults with disabilities being lonely, sedentary, cognitively vulnerable, and trusting of strangers make them targets of telephone scammers and telemarketers.

Another societal level influence is related to changes in gender-related roles that are occurring in many countries in an effort to achieve greater gender equality. These changes can lead to clashes between "traditionalists" and advocates for change; when these clashes take place within the family, they can lead to forms of domestic violence (Kosberg, 2014).

The Centers for Disease Control and Prevention (2014) cite societal level factors as a culture in which the following conditions occur:

- There is a high tolerance and acceptance of aggressive behavior.
- Family members are expected to care for elders without seeking help from others.
- There is little oversight over people in positions of authority who provide care for or make decisions about dependent older adults.
- Persons are encouraged to endure suffering or remain silent regarding their pains.
- There are negative beliefs about aging and elders.

In addition, Anetzberger (2013) states that emphasis on the acquisition of material things, which can lead to greed, can be a societal factor contributing to elder abuse.

SOCIAL ISOLATION AND LACK OF SOCIAL SUPPORT

Social isolation and lack of social support are closely related risk factors associated with many types of abuse. Social isolation can arise from the older adult, the perpetrator, or social circumstances, as in the following examples:

- Older adults may self-isolate as a means of maintaining privacy, autonomy, and control over their lives.

- Older adults may self-isolate to avoid the imposition of unwanted services.

- Older adults with dementia may self-isolate because of embarrassment, impaired decision-making abilities, or impaired ability to initiate actions and solve problems.

- Older adults who are depressed may self-isolate to avoid unwanted social interactions, even with family.

- Caregivers and family who engage in abusive behaviors may foster social isolation to avoid detection.

- Caregivers and family may use social isolation as a component of psychological abuse.

- Social isolation may be inherent in the geographic environment, for example, in rural areas.

- Communication barriers can lead to social isolation (e.g., being deaf, not speaking the dominant language).

- Cultural differences can lead to social isolation (e.g., being an immigrant).

Although social isolation is primarily a risk for elder abuse in domestic settings, it also applies to residents of long-term care facilities. For example, elder abuse is more likely to occur in the absence of visitors who advocate for individualized care and observe the care that is provided for residents who have dementia (Dayton, 2013). Even residents who do not have dementia may feel intimidated and need family advocacy to assure that their needs are met and they are honored and respected as individuals.

Members of minority and stigmatized groups experience social isolation in unique ways that can increase their vulnerability to elder abuse, as discussed in Chapter 5 in relation to cultural factors. Older adults who identify as lesbian, gay, bisexual, or transgender (LGBT) have a unique history of decades of oppression and prejudice and these circumstances increase their vulnerability to elder abuse as in the following examples:

- In domestic settings, partners may use "blackmail techniques" to deny care or exploit resources.

- In community settings, LGBT older adults often have a long-term pattern of social isolation because they lived most of their lives in secrecy.

- In institutional settings, staff who hold prejudices may use name-calling or make derogatory comments about LGBT residents.

- In any setting, LGBT older adults are vulnerable to any type of abuse by people who hold prejudices.

- Older gay men are vulnerable to abuse by younger gay men as well as by homophobic people.

Lack of social support as a risk for elder abuse can apply to both the vulnerable older adult who becomes a victim and the family caregivers who become perpetrators. Although lack of social support goes hand-in-hand with social isolation, it also has a broader societal aspect in that needed social supports may not be available for older adults or caregivers. In some situations, social support is available but barriers exist to the use of these services. When lack of information about available support services is a barrier, health care professionals can address this in clinical settings. Barriers that are more difficult to address include resistance to services on the part of the older adult and caregivers, and inaccessibility of acceptable, affordable, and appropriate programs on the part of society. Roles of nurses in addressing these barriers are discussed in Part III of this book.

> What if they find out I am a lesbian? . . . You have to stop being the person that you really are . . . you become isolated. . . . You're not yourself. (Walsh et al., 2011)

FACTORS ASSOCIATED WITH ELDER ABUSE BEING UNDETECTED AND UNREPORTED

As already noted, only a fraction of the known or suspected elder abuse cases are reported to authorities, and this is associated with risk factors at societal and situational levels. The most obvious risk factor at the situational level is that perpetrators are highly motivated to avoid detection. Victims try to avoid detection for a variety of reasons including fear, shame, denial, humiliation, relationship with abuser, and physical or cognitive inability to request help. In addition, social isolation is a risk not only for the occurrence of elder abuse but also for lack of detection. In domestic abuse by a family member, both the victim and the perpetrator may be influenced by the dominant ideology of familialism, which reinforces the notion of family as private, inviolable, and immune to dysfunctional processes (Norris, Fancey, Power, & Ross, 2013). Additional situational reasons that domestic elder abuse goes unreported include language and cultural barriers; perceived or actual lack of support resources; and a strong sense of self-reliance for solving problems without outside help on the part of the older adult, the caregiver, or both. Societal reasons include invisibility, lack of training about detection, lack of information about reporting, fear of harming relationships, and belief that professionals can resolve issues without protective services.

CONSEQUENCES OF ELDER ABUSE

Serious consequences are associated with elder abuse at both the personal and societal levels. On the personal level, abused older adults experience higher rates of stress, depression, and emotional trauma; lower levels of quality of life; and increased dependency on others. Perhaps most seriously, studies have found that elder abuse significantly increases the risk of dysfunction, disability, illness, and death (e.g., Dong, 2005; Dong et al., 2009, 2011).

Examples of consequences for individual older adults may include the following:

- Effects on overall health: increased risk for functional limitations, disability, increased risk for being admitted to an institutional setting
- Psychological/emotional effects: fear, anxiety, depression; decreased self-esteem; feelings of shame, guilt, powerlessness, self-blame
- Effects on longevity: shorter life span
- Social effects: isolation, depression, stigma
- Immediate effects of physical abuse: pain, burns, bruises, fractures, malnutrition, dehydration, life-threatening injuries, death
- Effects of financial abuse: loss of assets, inability to pay for basic care needs

■ Effects of sexual abuse: physical injury and trauma, especially to thighs, genitalia, and perineum; emotional trauma, including posttraumatic stress disorder; sexually transmitted diseases

Older people haven't the confidence to . . . fight back. If you were younger you probably could do something about it, but you get older and they make you lose your confidence and then you don't think you can do anything, no matter what you do. (Taylor et al., 2014, p. 230)

For several decades, legislators, gerontologists, and social service providers have discussed consequences of elder abuse from a societal perspective with attention more recently to implications related to health care services. For instance, a longitudinal study of nearly 10,000 community-living older adults in Chicago identified the following serious outcomes pertinent to health care services (Dong, 2013; Institute of Medicine and National Research Council, 2014):

■ Increased mortality rates from all causes (5.9 deaths/100 for those without elder abuse and 18.3 deaths/100 for abused older adults)

■ Greater use of emergency department services

■ Increased rates of hospitalizations

■ Increased use of and shorter length of stay in hospice

■ Increased rates of admission to nursing homes

WHY NURSES NEED TO KNOW ABOUT ELDER ABUSE

From a statistical perspective, nurses in adult health care settings could encounter elder abuse in at least 10% of situations in which they care for older adults. Most of these cases are not recognized as elder abuse and even fewer are reported to appropriate agencies. Health care practitioners are currently being called on to address elder abuse and neglect as a public health problem that demands urgent attention. "If a new illness were identified that affected so many older individuals, and for which risk was heightened further for vulnerable subpopulations, it would likely be considered a public health crisis. A similar sense of urgency is needed to ensure that older individuals are free from mistreatment" (Pillemer, Connolly, Breckman, Spreng, & Lachs, 2015, p. 321).

From a legalistic perspective, nurses need to know about elder abuse because nurses are required to report suspected—not necessarily verified—cases of elder abuse to appropriate authorities, as discussed in Chapter 6. From a personal perspective, most nurses can identify relatives, friends, or acquaintances who are or have been victims of abuse if they reflect on their experiences outside of their professional responsibilities.

Most importantly, from professional, humanistic, and ethical perspectives, nurses need to know about elder abuse so they can care holistically for older adults. Knowledge about types of elder abuse provides the foundation for recognizing that an older adult requires comprehensive care from multidisciplinary health professionals who can take actions to prevent abuse and address ongoing abuse. Nurses are in key positions to identify older adults who are at risk for or victims of elder abuse and to take leadership roles in addressing this serious and all-too-common but often unrecognized problem.

KEY POINTS: WHAT NURSES NEED TO KNOW AND CAN DO

- The seven types of elder abuse defined by the National Center on Elder Abuse are self-neglect, neglect, physical abuse, emotional (psychological) abuse, exploitation, sexual abuse, and abandonment.

- Causation of elder abuse is a complex phenomenon associated with risks within the older adult, perpetrator, relationship, and broader social environment (Box 1.1).

- Social isolation and lack of social support are risks that are associated with many types of abuse.

- Victims of elder abuse experience many serious consequences, including physical and psychological effects.

- Nurses have essential roles in identifying and addressing elder abuse when they care for older adults.

REFERENCES

Acierno, R., Hernandez-Tejada, M., Muzzy, W., & Steve, K. (2010). *National Elder Mistreatment Study*. Report to the National Institute of Justice (Project #2007-WG-BX-0009). Rockville, MD: National Institute of Justice.

Anetzberger, G. J. (2012). An update on the nature and scope of elder abuse. *Generations, 36*(3), 12–20.

Anetzberger, G. J. (2013, August 14). *Elder abuse risk factors* [Podcast, Part I]. National Center on Elder Abuse. Retrieved from www.ncea.aoa.gov/Resources/Webinar/index.aspx

Baker, A. (1975). Granny-battering. *Modern Geriatrics, 5*, 20–24.

Bowes, A., Ghizala, A., & Macintosh, S. B. (2012). Cultural diversity and the mistreatment of older people in Black and minority ethnic communities: Some implications for service provision. *Journal of Elder Abuse & Neglect, 24*, 251–274.

Burston, G. R. (1975). Granny-battering [Letter to the editor]. *British Medical Journal, 3* (5983), 592.

Butler, R. N. (1969). Ageism: Another form of bigotry. *Gerontologist, 9*, 243–246.

Butler, R. N. (1975). *Why survive? Being old in America.* New York, NY: Harper & Row.

Centers for Disease Control and Prevention. (2014). *Elder abuse: Risk and protective factors.* Retrieved from www.cdc.gov/violenceprevention/elder abuse/riskprotectivefactors.html

Daniel, B., & Bowes, A. (2011). Re-thinking harm and abuse: Insights from a lifespan perspective. *British Journal of Social Work, 41*, 820–836.

Dayton, C. (2013). *Elder abuse risk factors* [Podcast, Part I]. August 14, 2013. National Center on Elder Abuse. Retrieved from www.ncea.aoa.gov/ Resources/Webinar/index.aspx

Dong, X. (2005). Medical implications of elder abuse and neglect. *Clinics in Geriatric Medicine, 21*, 293–313.

Dong, X. (2013). Elder abuse: Research, practice, and health policy. The 2012 GSA Maxwell Pollack Award lecture. *Gerontologist, 54*, 153–162.

Dong, X., Chen, R., & Simon, M. (2014). Elder abuse and dementia: A review of the research and health policy. *Health Affairs, 33*(4), 642–649. doi:10 .1377/hlthaff.2013.1261

Dong, X., Simon, M., Beck, T., McCann, J., Farran, C., Laumann, E., . . . Evans, D. (2011). Elder abuse and mortality: The role of psychological and social wellbeing. *Gerontology, 57*, 549–558.

Dong, X., Simon, M., Mendes de Leon, C., Fulmer, T., Beck, T., Hebert, L., . . . Evans, D. (2009). Elder self-neglect and abuse and mortality risk in a community-dwelling population. *Journal of the American Medical Association, 302*, 517–526.

Harbison, J., Coughlan, S., Beaulieu, M., Karabanow, J., Vanderplaat, M., Wildeman, S., & Wexler, E. (2012). Understanding "Elder Abuse and Neglect": A critique of assumptions underpinning responses to mistreatment and neglect of older people. *Journal of Elder Abuse & Neglect, 24*, 88–103.

Hudson, M. (1991). Elder mistreatment: A taxonomy with definitions by Delphi. *Journal of Elder Abuse & Neglect, 3*(2), 1–20.

Institute of Medicine and National Research Council. (2014). *Elder abuse and its prevention: Workshop summary.* Washington, DC: National Academies Press.

Killick, C., Taylor, B. J., Begley, E., Carter-Anand, J., & O'Brien, M. (2015). Older people's conceptualization of abuse: A systematic review. *Journal of Elder Abuse & Neglect, 27*, 100–120.

Kosberg, J. I. (2014). Rosalie Wolf Memorial Lecture: Reconsidering assumptions regarding men as elder abuse perpetrators and as elder abuse victims. *Journal of Elder Abuse & Neglect, 26*, 207–222.

Lifespan of Greater Rochester, Inc., Weill Cornell Medical Center of Cornell University, & New York City Department for the Aging. (2011). *Under the radar: New York State Elder Abuse Prevalence Study*. New York, NY: Author.

Lithwick, M., Beaulieu, M., Gravel, S., & Straka, S. M. (2000). The mistreatment of older adults: Perpetrator-victim relationships and interventions. *Journal of Elder Abuse & Neglect, 11*(4), 95–112.

Mysyuk, Y., Westendorp, R., & Lindenberg, J. (2013). Added value of elder abuse definitions: A review. *Ageing Research Review, 12*, 50–57.

National Center on Elder Abuse. (n.d.). *Forms of elder abuse*. Retrieved from www.ncea.aoa.gov/Resources/Webinar/index.aspx

Naughton, C., Drennan, J., & Lafferty, A. (2014). Older people's perceptions of the term elder abuse and characteristics associated with a lower level of awareness. *Journal of Elder Abuse & Neglect, 26*, 300–318.

Norris, D., Fancey, P., Power, E., & Ross, P. (2013). The critical-ecological framework: Advancing knowledge, practice, and policy on older adult abuse. *Journal of Elder Abuse & Neglect, 25*, 40–55.

Pillemer, K., Connolly, M.-T., Breckman, R., Spreng, N., & Lachs, M. (2015). Elder mistreatment: Priorities for consideration by the White House Conference on Aging. *Gerontologist, 55*, 320–327.

Taylor, B. J., Killick, C., O'Brien, M., Begley, E., & Carter-Anand, J. (2014). Older people's conceptualization of elder abuse and neglect. *Journal of Elder Abuse & Neglect, 26*, 223–243.

Walsh, C. A., Olson, J. L., Ploeg, J., Lohfeld, L., & Macmillan, H. L. (2011). Elder abuse and oppression: Voices of marginalized elders. *Journal of Elder Abuse & Neglect, 23*, 17–42.

World Health Organization. (n.d.). *Elder abuse* (Fact sheet number 357). Retrieved from www.who.int/mediacentre/factsheets/fs357/en

2

ELDER ABUSE IN DOMESTIC SETTINGS BY A TRUSTED OTHER

Despite much public attention to elder abuse in nursing home settings, the reality is that 89.3% of reported elder abuse victims are older adults who live in their own homes or other private-care settings in the community (Teaster et al., 2006). This is due, at least in part, to the fact that 93% of older adults live in independent housing and an additional 3.5% live in independent settings that provide some assistance with daily care, with only 3.5% of older adults residing in nursing homes (Administration on Aging, 2013). In this and the next chapter, elder abuse in domestic settings is discussed from two perspectives: abuse involving a perpetrator (this chapter) and self-neglect and hoarding as aspects of domestic elder abuse that do not involve an outside perpetrator (Chapter 3).

OVERVIEW OF DOMESTIC ELDER ABUSE IN GENERAL

Domestic elder abuse occurs when a vulnerable older adult who lives in an independent setting (i.e., alone in his or her own home or with trusted others) is neglected, abused, or exploited by a trusted other. A *trusted other* is defined as a spouse/partner, friend, relative, neighbor, paid caregiver, family caregiver, or anyone on whom the older adult relies for support or assistance. There is an implicit or explicit expectation that the dependent person will receive adequate care from the person who is viewed as the caregiver. For example, spouses have a legal obligation to care for each other, and a few states require adult children to care for their parents. In addition, a duty to care is associated with a formal relationship (e.g., paid caregiver) or creating a reliance expectation.

Caregivers are often well intentioned; early in their caregiving role, they may provide good or even outstanding care. However, with increasing needs of the care recipient, the caregiver may become overwhelmed or lack the skills to provide good care. Other times, caregivers may experience functional or cognitive impairments and not only become incapable of providing care to others but also be in a position of needing care for themselves.

Because domestic elder abuse by a trusted other typically develops over months or years, it is often difficult to pinpoint an exact time at which it began. Domestic elder abuse by a trusted other who is a caregiver is particularly pertinent to nursing care of older adults for the following reasons:

- These situations often involve a combination of acute and chronic risk factors that can be addressed by health care professionals.
- Nurses are in key positions to identify risks for actual or potential domestic elder abuse.
- Nurses have key roles in working with family caregivers who are actual or potential perpetrators of elder abuse.
- Nursing interventions such as caregiver education or referrals to appropriate resources may be effective in preventing or resolving some situations of domestic elder abuse.

In contrast to abuse by trusted others, domestic abuse by strangers or acquaintances is associated with the unmet expectation that the older adult receives goods or services from sources who are honest and reliable. These situations, which are discussed as financial exploitation in Chapter 15, can occur either as one-time or short-term interactions or as repeated events over weeks, months, or years. When financial exploitation occurs in the context of trusted other relationships, these situations are often part of a broader picture that can include neglect, emotional abuse, physical abuse, or even sexual abuse.

Similar to financial exploitation, the perpetrator of sexual abuse can be either a trusted other or a stranger; however, the national prevalence study found that strangers comprised only 3% of perpetrators of sexual assault in domestic settings (Acierno, Hernandez-Tejada,

Muzzy, & Steve, 2009). Sexual abuse varies significantly from other types of abuse; it occurs across settings and by trusted others as well as strangers. This topic is addressed in Chapter 16.

Types of domestic elder abuse most commonly associated with a trusted other are described in this chapter in the context of characteristics of older adults, perpetrators, and their relationships. Although these aspects are discussed separately, every elder abuse situation involves complex interactions among the older adult and the perpetrator, and many situations involve several intertwined forms of abuse.

FORMS OF ELDER ABUSE BY TRUSTED OTHERS

Neglect, physical abuse, emotional abuse, and financial abuse by trusted others are discussed in this section because they occur commonly and are often interwoven. Manifestations of neglect and physical abuse can often be detected in clinical settings, but indicators of emotional and financial abuse are more nebulous. However, astute assessment skills can uncover clues and lead to interventions, as discussed in Parts II and III of this book. Brief case examples in this chapter provide an overview of types of abuse by trusted others and the unfolding case example in Chapter 12 illustrates roles of nurses in addressing domestic abuse.

Neglect

Neglect as a form of elder abuse is defined as "the refusal or failure by those responsible to provide food, shelter, health care or protection for a vulnerable elder" (National Center on Elder Abuse, n.d.). Responsibilities include, but are not limited to, the following: providing basic necessities of daily living, such as food and hydration; managing medications appropriately; addressing health care needs; attending to hygiene needs, including oral care; and maintaining a safe, stable, and comfortable living environment. Neglect can be active or passive, depending on whether the acts are of commission or omission.

Elder abuse scholars emphasize that neglect is a commonly reported form of elder abuse and is a potentially fatal syndrome associated with significant risk for morbidity and mortality (Fulmer & Dong, 2014). The National Elder Mistreatment Study identified low social support as the risk factor most strongly associated with potential neglect, with minority racial status, low income, and poor health as additional

CASE 2.1 Neglect by Trusted Other: Spouse

After Carlos Rodriguez retired, he cared for his wife, Marianna, in their home as her dementia progressed and she became increasingly confused and disoriented. Two months ago, Marianna forgot that they had moved and she began walking alone around the strange neighborhood looking for the church where she had attended daily services for nearly 40 years. Marianna does not dress appropriately for the weather and Carlos is rarely at home when the neighbors bring Marianna home.

CASE 2.2 Neglect by Trusted Other: Paid Caregiver

Sam Perkins lives alone and has moderate dementia. During the day, he attends a day-care center or is cared for by his family. Because he has a history of going outside, the family hired Sonia to provide social interaction when Sam is awake and to sit in the living room when he is sleeping. She is also expected to make sure he is safe at all times. Contrary to the agreement, Sonia sleeps soundly at night and the police frequently bring Sam home when they find him several blocks away, barefoot and wearing pajamas, despite the cold weather.

significant risk factors (Acierno et al., 2009). Neglect by trusted others can be intentional, unintentional, or both, depending on factors such as motivation, knowledge, and skill level of the responsible person. Also, neglect may evolve gradually as the health and functional levels of the caregiver or the older adult change. For example, a commonly encountered situation is that both older spouses develop dementia and attempt, unsuccessfully, to care for each other.

People who act as primary caregivers and live in the same household with, or provide care on a regular basis for, a vulnerable older adult can be held responsible for neglect as a form of elder mistreatment. If the person assumed to be responsible does not live in the same household, culpability is less clear. Perceptions of neglect and caregiving responsibilities can be strongly influenced by cultural factors (discussed in Chapter 5) and by societal and family expectations. In many situations, neglect develops gradually and health care professionals recognize it only after the effects are cumulative. For example, it is difficult to determine whether nutritional needs are being met until patterns of weight loss or clinical indicators of malnutrition are identified. In other situations, effects of neglect can be assessed within hours or days if the older adult has a medical condition that requires daily management. For example, an older adult with heart failure or insulin-dependent diabetes will experience immediate effects if the prescribed medical regimen is not followed.

Physical Abuse

Physical abuse is perhaps the most obvious type of domestic elder abuse, but even this type can be hidden and signs can be erroneously

CASE 2.3 Physical Abuse by Spouse

Jack Sanoma is relatively physically healthy but is unable to perform activities of daily living because of dementia. He has been married for 47 years to Evelyn, who provides all his care because she feels it is her duty. For the past year, Jack has been losing weight at the rate of about 3 lbs. a month, even though there is no medical reason for the weight loss. Evelyn does not use appropriate techniques to ensure that his nutritional needs are met and Jack is malnourished. Evelyn does not mind that Jack is losing weight because he has always been a large size and now it is easier to manage his care.

CASE 2.4 Physical Abuse by Nephew

Earl Zirkofski's Parkinson's has progressed to the point that he needs assistance with all daily activities. When Earl's nephew, Tom, lost his job and was on the verge of being homeless last year, he asked if he could move in and care for his "bachelor uncle." When Earl asks for assistance with getting into bed, Tom says his back is strained and he pushes his uncle onto the bed. One night Earl commented on the strong smell of alcohol on Tom's breath, and Tom punched him so hard that Earl fell to the floor.

attributed to other conditions. Any act that results in pain, discomfort, bodily injury, or functional impairment is considered physical abuse, as illustrated in the following wide array of examples:

- Hitting, slapping, pushing, kicking, shoving, burning, or striking with an object
- Causing falls and fall-related injuries
- Physical restraints, locking in confinement
- Inappropriate use of neuropsychiatric medications
- Withholding of medications necessary for comfort or control of medical conditions
- Excessive or forceful use of alcohol or other substances of abuse
- Force feeding, which can result in aspiration

Some of these examples overlap with other types of abuse or neglect. For example, depending on the intent, withholding of medications may be neglect and physical restraints may cause psychological abuse. At its worst, physical abuse includes shooting, strangulation, suffocation, and homicide.

The National Elder Mistreatment Study found that 76% of the perpetrators were family members. Characteristics of perpetrators at the time of the most recently reported physical mistreatment were as follows: 52% abusing substances, 36% unemployed, and 28% with history of treatment for mental illness. As with other forms of abuse, low social support for both the older adult and the perpetrator was strongly associated with an increased risk for physical mistreatment (Acierno et al., 2009).

Emotional/Psychological Abuse

The terms *emotional abuse* and *psychological abuse* are used interchangeably, although professional references tend to refer to psychological abuse and other references, including those citing perceptions of older adults, often refer to emotional abuse. Psychological abuse is difficult to identify and define because it is insidious, not readily observed, and highly influenced by cultural factors. For example, "there are fine lines and gray areas in the spectrum of normal bickering and name calling that develop into a pattern of psychological mistreatment, and physical, behavioral and social consequences are not as readily observable and attributable" (Conrad et al., 2011, p. 149). The National Center on Elder Abuse (n.d.) defines *psychological abuse* as the infliction of anguish, pain, or distress through verbal or nonverbal acts. Some elder abuse scholars distinguish between psychological abuse and psychological neglect. This is particularly pertinent in cultural contexts, as discussed in Chapter 5.

Psychological abuse often occurs in conjunction with other forms of elder abuse and it may be used as the means to an end, for example, to achieve financial gain. Another characteristic is that it involves a pattern of malicious and nonphysical acts calculated to create fear or undermine the victim's confidence and self-reliance. Examples of psychological abuse or neglect and the related abuser tactics include the following:

- Isolation: giving the "silent treatment," denying access to economic support; depriving the older adult of necessary aids and assistive devices, such as prosthetics, eyeglasses, walkers, or hearing aids; preventing contact with family or friends; preventing participation in previously enjoyed activities

- Insensitivity and disrespect: verbally insulting or humiliating, treating the older adult like a child, minimizing the older adult's injuries or complaints, not allowing the older adult to speak for himself or herself, intentionally disrespecting or disregarding cultural or religious values or practices of the older adult

- Shaming and blaming: yelling or swearing, willfully undermining the older adult's abilities to make decisions or remain independent for personal benefit, blaming the older adult for accidents, falsely claiming that an older adult has dementia

- Threats and intimidation: harassing the older adult, threatening or abusing the family pets, threatening nursing home placement, threatening harm to the older adult or loved ones, behaving in ways that frighten or intimidate the older adult (Conrad et al., 2011; National Center on Elder Abuse, 2013b).

The National Elder Mistreatment Study found that the risk for emotional abuse tripled for older adults with low social support and doubled for those who needed assistance with daily activities and in those with prior traumatic event experience. In addition, this study reported that half of the perpetrators of emotional abuse were unemployed and socially isolated, one fifth were abusing substances, and one fifth had some form of mental illness (Acierno et al., 2009). Even when emotional abuse is subtle, it can have a serious negative impact

---

CASE 2.5 Emotional Abuse by Son

Frank Amberston is 45 years old and moved back to his mother's house after his father died 15 years ago. Mrs. Amberston appreciates having a man around the house, especially since she began experiencing memory problems a few years ago. Her son receives monthly disability checks and is unemployed. Frank and his mother watch television together for 5 hours a day and in the evenings, Frank leaves a supply of wine near her chair before he goes out to the neighborhood bar. When Mrs. Amberston's daughters visit, they express concern about their mother's unkempt appearance, the spoiled food and garbage in the kitchen, dirty linens on the beds, smell of urine in the carpet, and overall messiness of the house. They also find hundreds of empty beer and wine bottles overflowing from waste baskets. They overhear Frank telling his mother that if he did not live there, she would be forced to go to a nursing home because she is "senile" and cannot take care of herself.

---

on the older person's emotional well-being. A study of older people's conceptualization of abuse and neglect found that "emotional abusiveness was viewed as underpinning all forms of abuse, and as influencing its experienced severity" (Taylor, Killick, O'Brien, Begley, & Carter-Anand, 2014, p. 223).

Financial Abuse

Financial abuse, which is also called financial exploitation, by a trusted other is defined as the illegal taking, misuse, or concealment of funds, property, or assets of a vulnerable elder (National Center on Elder Abuse, n.d.). Financial abuse can be deliberate and blatant, for example, when it entails blackmailing, forging the older adult's signature for financial gain, or transferring funds solely for use by another person. In other situations, however, it is less apparent as in the following examples:

- Inaccurate recording of financial transactions

- Promoting poor financial decisions

- Spending the older adult's money, ostensibly for the purpose of caring for the older adult

- Serving as representative payee for an older adult who is capable of overseeing his or her own financial matters
- Using the older adult's assets in exchange for care or services in a manner that is questionable or disproportionate
- Assuming ownership of the older adult's vehicles for personal use

Situations in which the older adult lives in the same household with a family member who provides care may involve mutual dependency including financial benefits for both parties. At the same time, questions often arise about financial exploitation by the family caregiver, such as the following:

- Does the adult child have an obligation to provide needed care for her parents?
- What financial gains or losses are involved for the dependent older adult?
- What financial gains or losses are involved for the family caregiver, either during the caregiving time or as inheritance?
- Does the family caregiver deserve compensation equal to what would be spent for care provided by others?
- Does the family caregiver use undue influence to gain assets that would be more than the fair value of services provided?
- Does one family member use undue influence to benefit unfairly in relation to siblings or other family members who would be entitled to equal compensation?

> Well I know for a fact that my brother robbed my mother blind, but my mother thought the sun shone on his backside . . . there is nothing you can do about it . . . as far as she was concerned she wasn't being abused. He was coming to visit her. (Taylor et al., 2014, p. 231)

These questions are addressed within the context of the older person's needs and abilities, the characteristics of the family caregiver who is actually or potentially an abuser, and the dynamics of the relationship between the older adult and the trusted other.

ENVIRONMENT FOR DOMESTIC ELDER ABUSE BY A TRUSTED OTHER

Situations of domestic elder abuse by a trusted other involve unique interconnections among three components: a vulnerable older adult, a

CASE 2.6 Financial Exploitation by Family

Anthony Smith moves in with his mother who has mild dementia. He transfers the house title to his name and withdraws large amounts of money from his mother's bank account. He drives her car, but does not take her to her usual social activities, such as church and the senior center. Mrs. Smith is afraid to say anything because she depends on her son for her care.

CASE 2.7 Financial Exploitation by Trusted Other

Carl paid his long-time neighbor Brenda to provide transportation, light housekeeping, grocery shopping, and meal preparation because he lived alone and was visually impaired. When Carl's macular degeneration progressed to the point that he could no longer write checks, he relied on Brenda to assist with banking and bill paying. Carl's son assisted him with his income tax and found that his bank account had been depleted. Also, the credit card that Brenda used at the gas station showed unusually high charges for the past 5 months.

perpetrator, and the relationship between the older adult and the perpetrator. Because relationship factors are the "glue" that connects the vulnerable older adult and the trusted other who becomes a perpetrator, each domestic elder abuse situation inherently involves a broken trust relationship. In addition, all elder abuse situations develop within the broader societal context, as discussed in Chapter 1. Social isolation and low social support are situational characteristics of particular importance to identifying and addressing elder abuse in clinical settings. Risks associated with each of these components can be viewed as the environment for domestic elder abuse by a trusted other, as illustrated in Figure 2.1.

Dependency on Others

Dependency on others is a characteristic associated with either or both the vulnerable older adult and the trusted other who becomes a

FIGURE 2.1 Environment for domestic elder abuse.

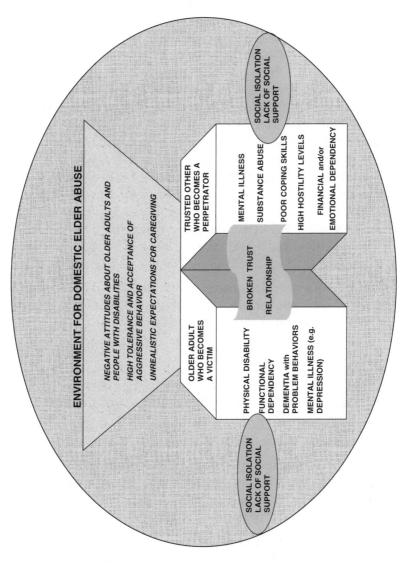

ENVIRONMENT FOR DOMESTIC ELDER ABUSE

NEGATIVE ATTITUDES ABOUT OLDER ADULTS AND
PEOPLE WITH DISABILITIES

HIGH TOLERANCE AND ACCEPTANCE OF
AGGRESSIVE BEHAVIOR

UNREALISTIC EXPECTATIONS FOR CAREGIVING

OLDER ADULT
WHO BECOMES
A VICTIM

PHYSICAL DISABILITY

FUNCTIONAL
DEPENDENCY

DEMENTIA with
PROBLEM BEHAVIORS

MENTAL ILLNESS (e.g.
DEPRESSION)

BROKEN TRUST
RELATIONSHIP

TRUSTED OTHER
WHO BECOMES A
PERPETRATOR

MENTAL ILLNESS

SUBSTANCE ABUSE

POOR COPING SKILLS

HIGH HOSTILITY LEVELS

FINANCIAL and/or
EMOTIONAL DEPENDENCY

SOCIAL ISOLATION
LACK OF SOCIAL
SUPPORT

SOCIAL ISOLATION
LACK OF SOCIAL
SUPPORT

33

perpetrator. Common forms of dependency in domestic elder abuse situations are emotional, functional, or financial or housing dependency. Although dependency on others does not necessarily lead to elder abuse, it can create a sense of powerlessness for the vulnerable older adult and foster fear of asking for help, particularly in combination with social isolation. For example, when dependency is mutual, the trusted other may take unfair advantage to meet his or her own needs and neglect or abuse the vulnerable older person. In many situations, emotional abuse is an integral component of controlling the dependent older adult and maintaining secrecy of the abusive situation.

Dependency of the older adult on the trusted other has traditionally been identified as a risk factor for elder abuse, but elder abuse scholars have also identified dependency needs of trusted others who become perpetrators. A summary of 21 studies published between 1988 and 2000 concluded that abusers tended to be dependent on their victims and were likely to have issues related to substance abuse, mental illness and depression, or cognitive impairments (Brandl & Cook-Daniels, 2002). Dependency of either or both the older adult or perpetrator influences domestic elder abuse situations in the following ways cited by Brandl and Cook-Daniels (2002):

- The dependency relationship may have started decades before it evolved into elder abuse, and it may have changed as the needs of the older adult or the trusted other changed.
- The victim and the abuser may benefit in tangible and intangible ways.
- Both the victim and the abuser may have reasons for maintaining their status quo, despite negative consequences for the older adult.
- These situations often occur within an environment of social isolation and low social support.
- The dependency relationship may increase resistance to outside help. When situations of domestic elder abuse are reported, most victims want to maintain the relationship while asking professionals to stop the abusive behavior.

In clinical settings, functional dependency needs of older adults are identified during assessments, but other types of dependency are more difficult to identify. Moreover, dependency needs of trusted others who actually or potentially mistreat the older adult are even more difficult to identify. Clues to dependency on the part of the abuser can be identified in certain characteristics of perpetrators such as substance abuse or diagnosis of mental illness. Shared housing is a type of dependency

CASE 2.8 Dependency on Others

Mrs. James experienced a renewed sense of having purpose in life when her alcoholic son, Thomas, moved back home after he told his mother that he had been "downsized" from his job but did not qualify for unemployment. Mrs. James had been a widow for 7 years and had developed an active social life but she was happy to have the companionship of her son. Thomas provides no care, takes financial advantage of her assets, and verbally abuses her when he is drunk. Mrs. James' two daughters have expressed concern about the living arrangement, but she tells them that if she continues to help Thomas, he will "stop drinking as soon as he gets a job again" and she will feel satisfied that she has been able to "save him." She expresses guilt about her husband's death from alcoholic cirrhosis and has always felt that Thomas would be there for her if she ever needed anything after her husband died. She tells her daughters that even though she is providing substantial financial assistance to Thomas, "things can be evened out after I die and I'm sure that Thomas will be sober by then."

that is often identified as a risk for elder mistreatment, even though it can be beneficial to both parties. Many times, the perpetrator is financially dependent on the older adult because of unemployment or patterns of excessive spending. Other times, the perpetrator has a sense of entitlement, particularly if he or she provides care for the older adult.

OLDER ADULT CHARACTERISTICS: FUNCTIONAL IMPAIRMENT AND MENTAL HEALTH ISSUES

A National Center on Elder Abuse (2013a) research brief cited evidence that adults with disabilities in community settings experience disproportionately higher rates of all types of abuse and triple the rate of serious violent crime compared with those without disabilities. Functional impairment and poor physical health are vulnerability characteristics for elder abuse in many ways. Most obviously, people with greater physical disability rely on others for even their most basic personal care needs. This dependency opens the door for caregivers to become perpetrators of elder abuse, either intentionally or unintentionally. Table 2.1 presents examples of functional limitations and

TABLE 2.1 Examples of Functional Limitations and Associated Risk for Elder Abuse

EXAMPLES OF FUNCTIONAL LIMITATION	ASSOCIATED RISK FOR ELDER ABUSE
Limited mobility	Difficulty escaping when safety is threatened; difficulty meeting basic needs
Mobility and balance problems	Increased susceptibility to falls and injuries when physically mistreated
Limitations with shopping, meal preparation, and eating	Increased risk for malnutrition and dehydration in the absence of appropriate resources and assistance
Confinement to bed or chair	Risk for pressure ulcers in the absence of appropriate care; risk for inadequate care
Swallowing difficulties	Risk for aspiration when consistency of food and fluid is inappropriate or when caregivers do not use correct techniques
Inability to self-administer pain medications	Risk for substitutes or smaller doses because the caregiver uses the medication or sells it to others
Needing assistance with financial management, ranging from simple bill paying to oversight of all assets	Risk for financial exploitation
Impaired decision making	Inability to seek help when needed; increased vulnerability to scams and financial exploitation

associated risks for elder abuse. Mental health issues are also associated with an increased risk for becoming a victim of elder abuse. Studies have found that depression, anxiety, loneliness, and lower levels of social relations increased the risk for elder abuse in community-dwelling older adults (Dong & Simon, 2014; Roepke-Buehler, Simon, & Dong, 2015).

Substance abuse can also be a mental health issue for victims of elder abuse in the following ways, as cited by the National Committee for the Prevention of Elder Abuse (n.d.):

- Substance abuse may contribute to cognitive impairments or emotional dependency and decrease the person's ability to resist or detect coercion or fraud.

- Substance abuse may contribute to physical disability and medical problems to increase the person's functional dependency.

- Perpetrators may encourage or even use force or coercion to promote excessive use of alcohol or drugs to make the victim more compliant or vulnerable.

- Victims may use drugs or alcohol as a coping mechanism to relieve anxiety or fear.

- Older adults who have a history of substance abuse or currently are substance abusers are likely to have poor or dysfunctional relationships with family and others on whom they depend for care.

Cognitively impaired older adults are at increased risk for elder abuse because they may not even recognize abuse or neglect and they are less able to provide self-care or protect themselves from abusers. Specific aspects of cognitive function that increase the risk for elder abuse include memory impairment, slowed thought processing, and poor executive function (i.e., decision-making skills; Ernst et al., 2014). Dementia is discussed in the next section as a mental health issue strongly associated with increased risk for elder abuse.

If you are living in the care of your own family and you are having abuse, you would be reluctant to report them or to say anything about it because you don't want to hurt them and at the same time you need the help, you probably even do not understand it's abuse. (Taylor et al., 2014, p. 230)

OLDER ADULT CHARACTERISTIC: DEMENTIA

Dementia is frequently identified as a risk for elder abuse, with studies reporting prevalence rates between 25% and 55%, and higher rates associated with minority groups and people with a history of intimate partner violence (Tronetti, 2014). Dementia increases the vulnerability of older adults to abuse in many ways, as in the following examples:

- Difficulty in managing personal finances increases the risk for financial exploitation, even during early stages when the older adult functions well in all or many other aspects.

- Cognitive impairments interfere with the ability of the older adult to perceive and self-report elder abuse.

- Dementia is associated with social isolation, which is a risk factor for elder abuse.

- When elder abuse is suspected, older adults with dementia may not be reliable sources of information, or their credibility may be questionable.

- Increased risk for abuse is associated with dementia-related behaviors during all stages, including anxiety, aggression, agitation, and neuropsychiatric manifestations.

- Functional dependency increases the risk for all types of abuse.

- Long-term and progressive course of dementia creates risk factors for all types of elder abuse.

CASE 2.9 Mild Dementia

Dorothy Hampton was diagnosed with mild dementia 18 months ago and lives with her husband, who has recently retired. As her short-term memory has become more impaired, she frequently asks her husband the same question repeatedly. He has become increasingly impatient with her repeated questions and told her that he would no longer answer the same question more than twice. When she asks the same question a third time, he tells her she is too stupid to talk to and he leaves the house or isolates her in the basement for an hour.

CASE 2.10 Dementia With Difficult Behaviors

Raymond lives with his son and daughter-in-law and attends a memory-care center every day when they are at work. In the evenings, Raymond often expresses fear of intruders and tells his son that strangers are looking through the windows and are planning to break in and rob them. Rather than addressing Raymond's anxiety with reassurance, his son gives him beer and sleeping pills. His son turns the lights off and stays in the same room playing loud video games on the big screen.

CASE 2.11 Dementia With Significant Functional Dependency

Harriett is 88 and moved to her granddaughter's house 3 years ago because her dementia had progressed. Her granddaughter is a stay-at-home single mother of four children, ages 4 to 10. Harriett requires significant assistance with all activities of daily living. During the past 18 months, she has been losing about 3 lbs. every month because the 10-year-old great granddaughter is supposed to assist her with meals but is always in a hurry. Harriett occasionally receives help from her granddaughter with a "sponge bath" but her hair has not been washed in 6 months and her toenails need to be cut.

Because the usual course of dementia is associated with different manifestations, risks for elder abuse differ significantly as the condition progresses, as illustrated in Cases 2.9, 2.10, and 2.11.

PERPETRATOR CHARACTERISTICS

A national study defining the scope of elder abuse found that almost 90% of trusted others who became perpetrators were family members, as illustrated in Figure 2.2. Alcohol or substance abuse is the perpetrator risk factor most consistently identified in studies of all forms and age groups of domestic abuse. Alcohol abuse is particularly strong as a perpetrator risk factor for physical or sexual abuse by spouses (Yon, Wister, Mitchell, & Gutman, 2014). A review of state-reported cases found a strong association between domestic elder abuse and perpetrator's use of marijuana and cocaine rather than alcohol (Jogerst, Daly, Galloway, Zheng, & Xu, 2012). Other perpetrator risks commonly identified include depression; diagnosis of mental illness; inadequate coping skills; financial pressures; high levels of general hostility or anger; and history of social, mental, and/or legal problems. Perpetrator risks associated with caregiving are discussed in the following section.

The old guy can get a little drunk so that it's easy to slap the old lady around. (Erlingsson, Saveman, & Berg, 2005, p. 217)

FIGURE 2.2 Perpetrators of domestic elder abuse.

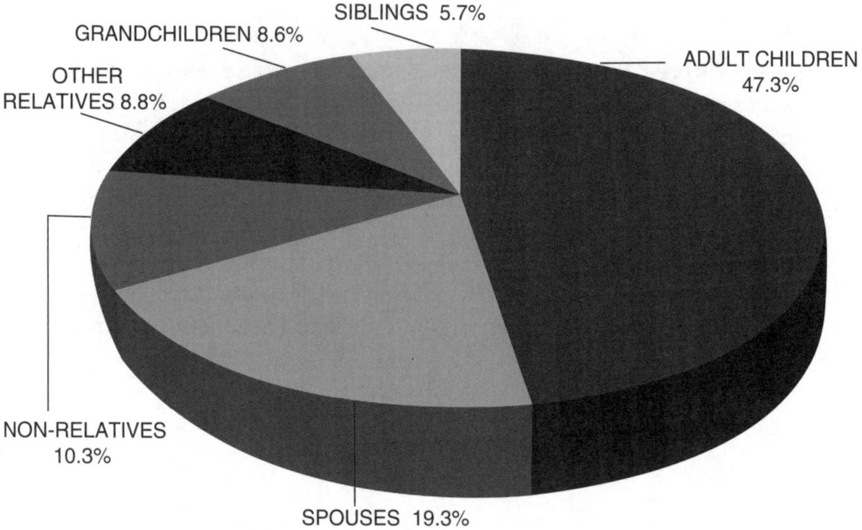

SIBLINGS 5.7%

GRANDCHILDREN 8.6%

OTHER RELATIVES 8.8%

ADULT CHILDREN 47.3%

NON-RELATIVES 10.3%

SPOUSES 19.3%

Adapted from Administration on Aging (1998).

RELATIONSHIP CHARACTERISTICS

Relationship characteristics are perhaps the most complex type of risk factors because they involve current and past (usually long-term) interactions between the older adult and the trusted other who becomes a perpetrator. Relationship characteristics may involve power and control issues or issues related to a history of violence within the family. Although numerous theories about elder abuse causation address relationship characteristics, this discussion focuses on two aspects that are most commonly addressed in clinical settings: caregiver factors and intimate partner violence. Mutual abuse, in which the victim directs abusive behaviors toward the perpetrator, also occurs within the context of relationships involving caregivers and intimate partners. In some cases, particularly those involving two people with dementia, the lines between victim and perpetrator are blurred or even overlap.

Caregiver Factors

Early studies of elder abuse focused on caregiver stress and burden as a major contributing factor to domestic elder abuse, but more recent studies do not support caregiver stress as a primary or sole reason for elder abuse (Brandl & Raymond, 2012). Current approaches do not discount the demands of long-term caregiving situations, particularly those involving families providing care for dependent older adults with progressive conditions such as dementia. Rather, the current emphasis is on identifying interacting conditions within the caregiving situation in combination with those within the broader community and societal settings that are associated with increased risk for elder abuse.

Studies have linked the following caregiver characteristics with increased risk of abusing the dependent older person: anxiety, depression, shared living, being a spouse, duration of caregiving, poor relationship prior to caregiving, and caregiver's perception of burden (Cooper, Blanchard, Selwood, Walker, & Livingston, 2010; Wiglesworth et al., 2010). A study of 417 caregivers who resided with the dependent older adult found that caregiver feelings of anger increase the risk for elder abuse, particularly when coupled with anxiety, depression, or resentment maltreatment (MacNeil et al., 2010). Other researchers suggested that caregivers who perceive high stress in caregiving and also have mental health issues or a history of substance abuse tend to attribute considerable power to the dependent older adult. When the dependent older adult does not comply with expectations, the caregiver becomes abusive to seek obedience (Lin & Giles, 2013).

> It's just the straw that breaks the camel's back. I would say stress, stress, and pressures. . . . The people that care the most [do the mistreating] because they always say that a good daughter is the one that bashes and the bad daughter walks away. (Bowes, Ghizala, & Macintosh, 2012, p. 266)

Intimate Partner Relationships

Situations involving abuse by a current or former spouse or intimate partner are considered *late-life domestic violence* or *intimate partner violence.* In most intimate partner violence situations, women are victims and men are perpetrators; however, it is important to recognize that men also are victims and women can be perpetrators. Many situations of late-life domestic violence initially involved bonds of love, caring, and attachment but developed into an abusive situation as the needs of one or both partner(s) changed. Other situations involve relationships that were marginally abusive during younger and middle adulthood but evolved into "domestic violence grown old," for example, if the couple became socially isolated and one or both developed dementia.

Explanations for intimate partner violence often center on traditional gender roles that emphasize a husband's authority and control
and a wife's obligation to obey. For older couples, these gender roles
may work well until one spouse is required to assume caregiving
responsibilities for the other. For example, one study of caregivers of
spouses with dementia found that older husbands tended to use
excessive force, coercion, or physical restraint when providing care;
however, women caregivers avoided aggressive strategies and experienced increased caregiver stress related to unresolved conflicts (Calasanti & King, 2007).

HOSPICE AND PALLIATIVE CARE IN HOME SETTINGS

Older adults receiving hospice or palliative care services in their home
settings can be vulnerable to abuse or neglect by trusted others because
these services often involve the administration of analgesic medications that could be used illegally and inappropriately by others. When
these services are provided in hospitals or nursing homes, there is professional accountability, including systems of checks and balances, for
the administration of medications. However, in home and residential
settings, there is little or no professional control over the administration of these medications and the recipient of services often relies on a
trusted other for access to analgesics. These situations create opportunities for caregivers to divert the analgesics for themselves or others by
withholding medications or replacing the prescribed medications with

CASE 2.12 Physical Abuse by Denying Medications

Ten years ago, Mr. and Mrs. Barker assumed custody of their grandson,
Dallas, because their daughter was addicted to heroin and their
son-in-law was in prison. Dallas, unemployed at age 20, continues to
live with his grandparents. Mr. Barker was recently diagnosed with
pancreatic cancer and receives hospice services at home. Because
Mrs. Barker has poor vision, she has not noticed that the hydromor-
phone (Dilaudid) has been replaced by a similar-looking vitamin.
Dallas suggests that his grandmother call the doctor to ask for a
stronger dose of the pain medication and he offers to go to the
drugstore for the new prescription.

a similar-looking substance. If nurses observe that pain medications are ineffective or are being refilled at shorter-than-expected intervals, it is important to consider the possibility that the older adult is not receiving the prescribed analgesic regimen. If the friends, family, or paid caregivers are abusing the drugs, this may be an elder abuse situation.

AVOIDING STEREOTYPES ABOUT ELDER ABUSE

It is important to recognize that some adults with many vulnerability characteristics do not become victims of elder abuse, just as some people with predisposing factors for cardiovascular disease do not experience a myocardial infarction. Older adults with vulnerability characteristics usually do not become victims of domestic elder abuse if their needs are addressed by reliable and honest caregivers in a supportive and appropriate social and physical environment. For example, an alcoholic nephew living with his aunt who has dementia may provide good care and not take advantage of the situation. Thus, nurses need to be on high alert for risks of elder abuse but not jump to conclusions when risk factors are present. In contrast, it is important to recognize that elder abuse occurs even in the absence of identifiable risk factors, as illustrated in Case 2.13.

CASE 2.13 Financial Exploitation Without Identifiable Risk Factors

Grace lives alone in a condominium and enjoys her newfound freedom after caring for her husband for the past 5 years until he died 6 months ago. She attends grief support groups and has returned to her volunteer activities delivering meals on wheels. Her granddaughter, Trudy, visits frequently and notices that the phone usually rings several times while she is there. After one of these calls, Grace says, "I'm not supposed to tell anyone about this, but since you overheard the call, I'll share with you that I've been dipping into the money that Harold left for me because I'm a big winner now. I'm sending one more cashier check for $5,000 and then I'll receive a million dollars from the lottery and a fancy car. Any taxes on the winnings are covered by the money I've already sent and this last installment is for processing the taxes and title for the car. They even told me I can pick the color of the car, so I chose silver blue."

Another aspect of avoiding stereotypes concerns assumptions about gender as a characteristic of either the victim or perpetrator. Although many references suggest that women are more likely to be victims and men are more likely to be perpetrators, studies indicate that this does not necessarily hold true. Kosberg (2014) reviewed this topic and cited the following research findings that are pertinent to domestic elder abuse:

- Abuse of older men is especially invisible and underreported, compared with abuse of older women

- Groups of older men particularly vulnerable to abuse include those having high-risk lifestyles and living in high-risk social settings (e.g., gay men, inner-city or rural settings, homeless or living alone)

- Older men who live in family settings and are vulnerable because of "retribution" by spouses, adult children, or other family members (e.g., related to abusive behavior decades earlier)

- Older men being reported as abusers, when, in fact, they are victims engaging in self-defense

CASE 2.14 Older Man Seeking Companionship

Maria Kirschenbacher and Harry Culpepper have been "companions" for 7 years, sharing a household, traveling together, and attending social events when they are invited by either family. Harry's family is concerned about the major income disparities related to Harry having substantial assets and Maria being entitled only to minimal Social Security income. In addition, they dislike the fact that Harry and Maria spend every winter in Harry's condominium in Arizona and never invite family to visit. After Harry developed macular degeneration and also began having memory problems, Maria took over all responsibility for driving and financial management. Last spring, when it was time to return home from Arizona, Harry called his son and asked him to pick him up at the airport because Maria was not coming back with him. When Harry's son called Maria, she told him that Harry is too forgetful and needs more care than she can provide. Upon investigation, Harry's family found out that the title to the condominium had been transferred to Maria's name. Harry told his family that, "that was the least I could do to provide for her because she has been so good to me."

Analysis of data from the National Elder Mistreatment Study found several key gender differences according to the type of mistreatment. For example, perpetrators of physical mistreatment against older men were more likely to be unemployed and have a history of legal problems (Amstadter et al., 2011).

Examples in this chapter underscore the importance of recognizing that risk factors can be "red flags" for detecting elder abuse but each elder abuse situation develops from a unique combination of factors that result in a broken relationship between a vulnerable older adult and a trusted other who becomes a perpetrator.

KEY POINTS: WHAT NURSES NEED TO KNOW AND CAN DO

- Domestic elder abuse situations are associated with risk and vulnerability factors in the older adult, trusted other, relationship between them, and environment (Figure 2.1).

- Types of domestic elder abuse most often encountered in health care settings include neglect, physical abuse, psychological abuse, and financial abuse.

- When nurses identify "red flags" for domestic elder abuse, they need to assess the overall situation, report suspected cases, and implement interventions.

REFERENCES

Acierno, R., Hernandez-Tejada, M., Muzzy, W., & Steve, K. (2009). *National Elder Mistreatment Study.* Report to the National Institute of Justice (Project #2007-WG-BX-0009). Rockville, MD: National Institute of Justice.

Administration on Aging. (1998). *National Elder Abuse Incidence Study.* Retrieved from aoa.gov/AoA_Programs/Elder_Rights/Elder_Abuse/Index.aspx

Administration on Aging. (2013). *Living arrangements of persons 65+, 2013.* Retrieved from www.aoa.gov/Aging_Statistics/Profile/2013/6.aspx

Amstadter, A. B., Cisler, J. M., McCauley, J. L., Hernandez, M. A., Muzzy, W., & Acierno, R. (2011). Do incident and perpetrator characteristics of elder mistreatment differ by gender of the victim? Results from the National Elder Mistreatment Study. *Journal of Elder Abuse & Neglect, 23*(1), 43–57.

Bowes, A., Ghizala, A., & Macintosh, S. B. (2012). Cultural diversity and the mistreatment of older people in Black and minority ethnic communities: Some implications for service provision. *Journal of Elder Abuse & Neglect, 24,* 251–274.

Brandl, B., & Cook-Daniels, L. (2002). *Domestic abuse in later life: A research review*. Retrieved from www.ncea.aoa.gov/Resources/Publication/docs/rschart.pdf

Brandl, B., & Raymond, J. A. (2012). Policy implications of recognizing that caregiver stress is not the primary cause of elder abuse. *Generations, 36*(3), 32–39.

Calasanti, T., & King, N. (2007). Taking "women's work" "like a man": Husbands' experiences of care work. *Gerontologist, 47*(4), 516–527.

Conrad, K. J., Iris, M., Ridings, J. W., Rosen, A., Fairman, K. P., & Anetzberger, G. J. (2011). Conceptual model and map of psychological abuse of older adults. *Journal of Elder Abuse and Neglect, 23*, 147–168.

Cooper, D., Blanchard, M., Selwood, A., Walker, Z., & Livingston, G. (2010). Famiy carers' distress and abusive behaviour: Longitudinal study. *British Journal of Psychiatry, 196*, 480–485.

Dong, X., & Simon, M. (2014). Vulnerability risk index profile for elder abuse in community-dwelling population. *Journal of the American Geriatrics Society, 62*, 10–15.

Erlingsson, C. I., Saveman, B.-I., & Berg, A. C. (2005). Perceptions of elder abuse in Sweden: Voices of older persons. *Brief, Treatment and Crisis Interventions, 5*(2), 213–227.

Ernst, J. S., Ramsey-Klawsnik, H., Schillerstrong, J. E., Dayton, C., Mixson, P., & Counihan, M. (2014). Informing evidence-based practice: A review of research analyzing adult protective services data. *Journal of Elder Abuse & Neglect, 26*, 458–494.

Fulmer, T. T., & Dong, X. (2014). Elder neglect: The state of the science. In Institute of Medicine and National Research Council. *Elder Abuse and Its Prevention: Workshop Summary* (pp. 67–74). Washington, DC: National Academies Press.

Jogerst, G. J., Daly, J. M., Galloway, L. J., Zheng, S., & Xu, Y. (2012). Substance abuse associated with elder abuse in the United States. *American Journal of Drug & Alcohol Abuse, 38*, 63–69.

Kosberg, J. (2014). Rosalie Wolf Memorial Lecture: Reconsidering assumptions regarding men as elder abuse perpetrators and as elder abuse victims. *Journal of Elder Abuse & Neglect, 26*, 207–222.

Lin, M. C., & Giles, H. (2013). The dark side of family communication: A communication model of elder abuse and neglect. *International Psychogeriatrics, 25*, 1275–1290.

MacNeil, G., Kosberg, J., Durkin, D., Dooley, W. K., DeCoster, J., & Williamson, G. M. (2010). Caregiver mental health and potentially harmful caregiving behavior: The central role of caregiver anger. *Gerontologist, 50*, 76–86.

National Center on Elder Abuse. (n.d.). *Forms of elder abuse*. Retrieved from www.ncea.aoa.gov/Resources/Webinar/index.aspx

National Center on Elder Abuse. (2013a). *Abuse of adults with a disability* [Research brief]. Retrieved from www.ncea.aoa.gov

National Center on Elder Abuse. (2013b). *NCEA elder abuse presentation: Psychological abuse*. Retrieved from www.ncea.aoa.gov

National Committee for the Prevention of Elder Abuse. (n.d.). *Elder abuse and substance abuse*. Retrieved from http://preventelderabuse.org/elder abuse/issues/substance.html

Roepke-Buehler, S. K., Simon, M., & Dong, X. (2015). Association between depressive symptoms, multiple dimensions of depression, and elder abuse: A cross-sectional, population-based analysis of older adults in urban Chicago. *Journal of Aging and Health, 27*(6), 1003–1025.

Taylor, B. J., Killick, C., O'Brien, M., Begley, E., & Carter-Anand, J. (2014). Older people's conceptualization of elder abuse and neglect. *Journal of Elder Abuse & Neglect, 26*, 223–243.

Teaster, P., Dugar, T., Mendiondo, M., Abner, E., Cecil, K., & Otto, J. (2006). *The 2004 survey of state adult protective services: Abuse of adults 60 years of age and older*. Washington, DC: National Center on Elder Abuse.

Tronetti, P. (2014). Evaluating abuse in the patient with dementia. *Clinics in Geriatric Medicine, 30*, 825–838.

Wiglesworth, A., Mosqueda, L., Mulnard, R., Liao, S., Gibbs, L., & Fitzgerald, W. (2010). Screening for abuse and neglect of people with dementia. *Journal of the American Geriatrics Society, 58*, 493–500.

Yon, Y., Wister, A., Mitchell, B., & Gutman, G. (2014). A national comparison of spousal abuse in mid- and old age. *Journal of Elder Abuse & Neglect, 26*, 80–105.

ELDER ABUSE IN DOMESTIC SETTINGS: SELF-NEGLECT

In 1966, two British physicians applied the term *senile breakdown syndrome* to describe "a group of individuals who cease to maintain the standards of cleanliness and hygiene which are accepted by their local community" (Macmillan & Shaw, 1966, p. 1032). In the United States around that same time, the term *social breakdown syndrome* was used to describe behavioral manifestations of squalor, neglect of hygiene and personal environment, and refusal of assistance (Gruenberg, Brandon, & Kasius, 1966). Currently in the United States, self-neglect is considered a unique form of elder abuse, even though these situations rarely involve "abuse" per se and they also occur in younger adults.

During the past several decades, nurses, physicians, and other health care professionals have addressed self-neglect in many ways, including as a nursing diagnosis and a geriatric syndrome. This chapter describes self-neglect as a unique type of elder abuse with emphasis on aspects that are most relevant to addressing the needs of self-neglecting older adults in health care settings. Ethical issues related to self-neglect are addressed in Chapter 8, and aspects of nursing assessment and interventions are discussed in Chapters 9 and 10. Chapter 13 presents an unfolding case example illustrating responsibilities of nurses in addressing self-neglect in clinical practice.

DEFINITIONS AND SCOPE OF SELF-NEGLECT

The National Adult Protective Services Association (n.d.) defines *self-neglect* as "self-care and living conditions that are potentially hazardous to the health, safety or well-being of adults." This is one of at least 10 widely recognized definitions that typically include the following key concepts:

- Persistent lack of essential self-care (e.g., inattention to personal hygiene, seriously unkempt appearance)
- Persistent lack of cleanliness in the personal environment
- Lack of essential services and social support
- Personal behaviors that can lead to endangerment

In general, *self-neglect* is an umbrella term applied to a broad range of situations that involve a combination of personal behaviors and conditions within the person's environment that are actually or potentially harmful to the person or others. On the individual level, self-neglect includes a broad spectrum of health-related and self-care behaviors, ranging from nonadherence to health promotion recommendations at one end to self-abusive and life-threatening behaviors at the most serious end. On the environmental level, self-neglect situations range from minor disrepair of housing to squalor and life-endangering conditions, such as fire hazards and disease-promoting infestations. In communities, self-neglect is a major concern when the situation threatens the health and safety of others.

The majority of self-neglecting older adults live alone, but self-neglect can occur when two or more people live in unsafe conditions and have unmet needs for basic care. For example, an older couple who both have dementia may live unsafely in self-neglecting conditions in their own home. Self-neglect also applies to caregivers who neglect their health needs because they devote their time and energy to caring for someone else. In addition, elder abuse scholars currently are addressing the occurrence of self-neglect in semi-independent settings, such as assisted living facilities.

SELF-NEGLECT AS A UNIQUE FORM OF ELDER ABUSE

Although self-neglect is not defined specifically in all state elder abuse statutes, adult protective service agencies in all states accept referrals and investigate self-neglect. In reality, self-neglect is the most frequently encountered form of elder abuse addressed by adult protective service agencies. Manifestations of self-neglect are similar to those of neglect by caregivers; however self-neglect occurs in the absence of identifiable caregivers. Box 3.1 summarizes commonalities and differences between self-neglect and other forms of domestic elder abuse.

BOX 3.1   Self-Neglect and Other Forms of Domestic Elder Abuse: Commonalities and Differences

Common characteristics of self-neglect and other forms of domestic elder abuse

- Social isolation is often a contributing factor.
- The situation can develop either intentionally or unintentionally.
- A vulnerable older adult is perceived as needing protection from self or others.
- The older adult is perceived as needing assistance and lacking reliable and appropriate support services.
- Questions arise about the capacity of the older adult to accept or refuse assistance.
- Cultural norms of society affect perceptions of and approaches to the situations.
- Reported cases represent only the "tip of the iceberg" of suspected actual cases.
- If the situation does not pose threats to others, such as family, neighbors, or bystanders, it is more difficult to impose services.

Characteristics unique to self-neglect

- The danger of harm arises from the individual rather than from outsiders.
- Caregivers are not available as acceptable resources.
- Most self-neglecters do not perceive problems within their situation.
- Protective services can be imposed more readily when the person is being victimized by another person.
- Imposition of services changes the person's independence and threatens the right to be autonomous, independent, and to live in any chosen lifestyle.

RISK FACTORS FOR SELF-NEGLECT

Self-neglect occurs within the context of interactions among several risk factors in the older adult and his or her social and physical environments. Typically, older adults who become self-neglecting experience a combination of (a) physical disability or medical conditions, (b) cognitive impairments or mental illness, and (c) inadequate social supports. Specific health conditions identified as risks for self-neglect include diabetes, arthritis, dementia, depression, cardiovascular disorders, nutritional frailty, and bladder/bowel incontinence (Dyer, Goodwin, Pickens-Pace, Burnett, & Kelly, 2007; Ernst & Smith, 2011). Decline in physical function is associated not only with an increased risk for but also with greater seriousness of self-neglect (Dong et al., 2010). Elder abuse scholars increasingly are focusing on cognitive skills related to executive function as a condition that underlies all or most self-neglect situations, as discussed in the next section. Some psychosocial conditions associated with self-neglect include alcoholism, poor family relationships, and experiences of loss, grief, or abandonment. Table 3.1 lists some of the conditions in older adults that are associated with increased risk for self-neglect.

> Alcoholic . . . drank all my life . . . you couldn't get in or out, empty beer cans all over the place . . . used to accumulate . . . sold my saxophone for drink years ago. (Day, Leahy-Warren, & McCarthy, 2013, p. 84)

As with other types of elder abuse, social isolation and lack of social supports create risks for self-neglect. Social isolation occurs partially because self-neglecting older adults are likely to live alone and have little contact with family or friends. Lack of social supports occurs when the older adult does not use available services or when services are not available. Although self-neglecting older adults are often described as refusing services or resisting care, lack of care is sometimes rooted in the person's inability to perceive his or her own needs, as is common in these situations. In other situations, the person does recognize the need and would be willing to accept services, but acceptable services are not available. Analysis of data from adult protective service cases in Texas concluded that a lack of public social and health care services is a major risk for self-neglect, particularly in poor rural areas (Choi, Kim, & Asseff, 2009). These situations may be most amenable to resolution if service providers, including health care professionals, can identify acceptable social supports, as discussed in Chapter 11.

TABLE 3.1 Conditions That Increase the Risk for Self-Neglect

OLDER ADULT CONDITION	RELATED RISK FOR SELF-NEGLECT
Physical disability or impairment	Decreased ability to care for self and personal environment
Progressive or complex medical conditions	Potential for poor management leading to worsening of conditions (e.g., unmanaged hypertension leading to stroke)
Vision or hearing impairment	Social isolation, diminished ability to care for self and personal environment
Depression	Low self-esteem, lack of motivation, social isolation, decreased interest in self-care, self-harm, or suicidal thoughts or actions
Dementia	Cognitive changes affecting memory and executive function gradually affect all aspects of self-care and ability to remain independent
Stressful major life event	Grief, depression, social isolation
Excessive use of alcohol	Cognitive impairment, depression, malnutrition, self-injury, social isolation, nonadherence to medical care, avoidance of medical care to avoid detection
Anxiety disorders	Social isolation, phobias, difficulty adjusting to change
Delusions or paranoia due to mental illness	Social isolation, increased resistance to assistance, lack of insight, hoarding behaviors, distrust of outsiders, avoidance of medical care
Loss of familiar caregivers	Grief, depression, resistance to using new or outside resources
Low income status	Lack of financial resources for services
Low health literacy	Difficulty managing medical care

COGNITIVE CHARACTERISTICS IN RELATION TO SELF-NEGLECT

Cognitive characteristics of self-neglecting older adults need to be considered from two perspectives: (a) as conditions that increase the risk for self-neglect, and (b) as a major consideration with regard to the older adult's capacity for self-determination and right to refuse services. Ethical concerns are associated with cognitive and mental health characteristics because self-neglect situations typically involve questions about the older adult's capacity for self-care and self-protection and both of the following conditions also exist: (a) The person requires assistance with meeting basic needs, and (b) essential and acceptable supports are not being provided. When services are offered but the person refuses to accept them, ethical issues must be addressed in relation to the person's right to live in whatever way he or she chooses, regardless of consequences for the individual.

Cognitive Deficits as a Risk for Self-Neglect

Executive function has been identified as the cognitive skill that is most strongly correlated with self-care abilities of older adults referred to adult protective services for self-neglect (Schillerstrom et al., 2013). Executive function refers to a cluster of "master" cognitive processes that control, regulate, and manage all other cognitive processes. In everyday life, these processes help people focus attention, form goals, plan actions, self-monitor, solve problems, make decisions, and initiate and carry out goal-directed behaviors. A small degree of executive dysfunction is normal for all adults, both chronically and under stressful conditions. For example, under distracting conditions, it is usual to have difficulty focusing attention on tasks at hand. More serious degrees of executive dysfunction are often associated with pathologic conditions, such as dementia, depression, Parkinson's disease, and mental illnesses. Executive dysfunction can also be caused by medical conditions, including treatable ones, such as nutritional deficiencies. Table 3.2 summarizes manifestations of executive dysfunction that can lead to self-neglect, particularly in people who live alone and do not have adequate support resources.

Cognitive Function in Relation to Capacity to Refuse Services

Determination of a person's capacity to refuse services is based on a comprehensive assessment of cognitive skills related to decision making, as reviewed in detail in Chapter 9. In self-neglect situations,

TABLE 3.2 Executive Dysfunction as a Risk for Self-Neglect

MANIFESTATION OF EXECUTIVE DYSFUNCTION	EXAMPLE IN DAILY LIFE AS A RISK FOR SELF-NEGLECT
Inability to plan a task	Not shopping for groceries necessary for food preparations
Difficulty initiating a task	Not engaging in personal care activities, such as bathing or grooming
Poor problem solving	Repeatedly falling in a cluttered environment but not removing obstacles
Difficulty organizing information	Having bills and papers piled in numerous places and not knowing how to sort them
Inability to adapt to changing conditions	Living in a very cold environment and not figuring out who to call to fix the furnace
Impaired working memory	Not taking medications or going to medical appointments
Impaired self-monitoring	Driving a car unsafely
Impulsivity (i.e., impaired ability to think before acting)	Walking outside without being dressed appropriately for the weather

the assessment focuses on the person's abilities related to self-care and self-protections with emphasis on whether the person understands his or her circumstances and accepts appropriate steps to correct problems (Reyes-Ortiz, Burnett, Flores, Halphen, & Dyer, 2014). Box 3.2 presents key points of a brief checklist for determining capacity in self-neglect situations, which was developed by the Texas Elder Abuse and Mistreatment Institute (Reyes-Ortiz et al., 2014). This is not a substitute for a comprehensive assessment, but can be used as a screening tool in clinical settings.

If [you] infringe on [our] dignity . . . it's a difficult balance. Hopefully it's not a rat-ridden house or whatever. There are extremes that somebody will have to intervene, but I think sometimes people rush in and think "What's best for this lad; oh, residential care!" They don't sit down and ask "What do you think?" (Taylor, Killick, O'Brien, Begley, & Carter-Anand, 2014, p. 234)

BOX 3.2 Checklist for Determining Capacity in Self-Neglect Situations

Does the Person Understand His or Her Circumstances?

Despite adequate resources, the person . . .

_____   fails to perform an ADL* . . .

_____   fails to perform an IADL** . . .

_____   is exposed to an unsafe, unsanitary, or inadequate housing condition . . .

_____   has suffered abuse, neglect, exploitation, or self-neglect . . .

. . . and does not understand this fact

Is the Person Failing to Self-Care and Self-Protect?

Despite adequate resources, the person . . .

_____   is failing to perform an ADL . . .

_____   is failing to perform an IADL . . .

_____   is exposed to an unsafe, unsanitary, or inadequate housing condition . . .

_____   has suffered abuse, neglect, exploitation, or self-neglect . . .

. . . and does not take appropriate steps to correct the problem

*ADL, activity of daily living: toileting, dressing, grooming, ambulation, bathing.

**IADL, instrumental activity of daily living: shopping, food preparation, housekeeping, laundry, taking medications appropriately, using a telephone, arranging for transportation, handling finances.

Adapted from John M. Halphen for the Texas Elder Abuse and Mistreatment Institute, published in Reyes-Ortiz, Burnett, Flores, Halphen, and Dyer (2014).

Used with permission of Elsevier.

CHARACTERISTICS OF ENVIRONMENTS ASSOCIATED WITH SELF-NEGLECT

Self-neglect typically occurs in a personal environment of negligent and often unsanitary or even dangerous conditions. When conditions in the living space, house, and exterior surroundings are so unsanitary that they pose a danger to the health or safety of the occupant or others, the term *squalor-dwelling* is used (Aamodt, Terracina, &

Schillerstrom, 2015). Iris, Conrad, and Ridings (2014) developed an evidence-based scale for indicators of self-neglect, including clusters associated with physical and personal living conditions. Box 3.3 summarizes some of these indicators in the context of considerations related to environments.

HOARDING AS AN ASPECT OF SELF-NELGECT

Although many people lightly refer to "hoarding" when they stock their shelves with extra groceries or purchase duplicate items that are

---

BOX 3.3 Questions to Consider When Assessing the Environment in Relation to Self-Neglect

Does the Personal Environment . . .

. . . have evidence that the older adult is eating spoiled food?

. . . have odors or substances that raise concerns (e.g., urine, garbage, spoiled food, human or animal feces, vermin)?

. . . have an accumulation of garbage or items that presents a safety hazard?

. . . lack access to safe, sanitary, and operable toileting and bathing facilities?

. . . lack safe and operable supplies and equipment for food preparation (e.g., stove, refrigerator, sink with running water)?

. . . have risks for fire hazards or lack smoke detectors?

. . . have evidence of hoarding?

. . . lack at least one clear path for emergency evacuation?

. . . have pets that are excessive in numbers or not maintained?

. . . lack adequate lighting?

. . . lack a functional telephone?

. . . lack the ability to maintain a safe and comfortable temperature?

. . . lack basic functional utilities?

Adapted from Iris, Conrad, and Ridings (2014).

not needed immediately, in the context of a clinical diagnosis, hoarding is characterized by the following:

- Persistent difficulty discarding or parting with possessions, regardless of the value others may attribute to these possessions

- The accumulation of a large number of possessions that fill up and clutter active living areas of the home or workplace to the extent that their intended use is no longer possible

- The presence of significant personal distress or impairment in social, occupational, or other important areas of functioning

- Lack of insight

- Little or no motivation for change

- Difficulty or impossibility in maintaining a safe environment for self and others

Hoarding behaviors may occur as a manifestation of mental illnesses, such as schizophrenia or obsessive-compulsive disorder, in which cases the behaviors typically begin during early adulthood and gradually become more disabling. In older adults who become self-neglecting, hoarding behaviors are often associated with dementia or late-life depression. In these situations, the hoarding behaviors may arise from deficits in executive function that affect organizational abilities and awareness, as described in Table 3.2. Hoarding behaviors can lead to health problems and unsafe conditions, such as risks for falls and fires. Additional consequences that commonly occur in self-neglect situations include impaired daily functioning, food contamination, unsanitary environment, social isolation, impaired quality of life, and high levels of family frustration.

> I still have it because I haven't had the time to sort it out . . . I have a whole bunch here on the top shelf there that I want to get put away, . . . I like to get things straight. I am sorting things out. I am trying to get the order right. (Andersen, Raffin-Bouchal, & Marcy-Edwards, 2013, p. 445)

Animal hoarding is described as a public health problem characterized by a combination of the following conditions:

- The possession of more than the typical number of companion animals

- The inability to provide basic care, which can lead to illness, starvation, and death of the animals

- Denial about one's inability to provide care
- Lack of insight about the effects of the situation on the occupants, animals, and household environment (Patronek, 1999)

As with other types of hoarding, animal hoarding is a chronic condition that may progress from mild to severe. Adult protective service agencies cite compelling evidence of a strong association between animal hoarding and self-neglect by the animal hoarder (Nathanson, 2009). In contrast to object-hoarding environments, the vast majority of animal-hoarding households usually involve squalor and major personal and public health hazards (Frost, Patronek, & Rosenfield, 2011).

PERSPECTIVES OF OLDER ADULTS WHO BECOME SELF-NEGLECTERS

Qualitative studies of older adults identified as hoarders or self-neglecters provide insight into the broader social aspects of self-neglecting older adults. For example, a dominant theme identified through interviews with 16 self-neglecting elders in Israel is that their current conditions of self-neglect were "anchored in cumulative experiences of frequent transitions, the inability to put down roots, a sense of isolation, attempts to acclimatize and to survive alongside personal losses and traumatic life circumstances" (Band-Winterstein, Doron, & Naim, 2012, p. 113). Box 3.4 describes perspectives of five older adults identified as self-neglecting. Similarly, interviews with eight self-neglecting older adults in Ireland identified common experiences of multiple hardships during early life, along with themes of social isolation, vulnerability, frugality, and service refusal (Day et al., 2013).

AVOIDING STEREOTYPES ABOUT SELF-NEGLECTING OLDER ADULTS

As with other types of elder abuse, it is imperative to avoid stereotypes. This is particularly pertinent with regard to the older adult's acceptance of services. When service providers and health care professionals encounter a self-neglect situation, they may be inclined to judge the person as noncompliant and resistant. Many times, however, self-neglecting older adults lack awareness of their situation due to cognitive impairments and they are receptive to interventions if

BOX 3.4 Older Adults Describe the Life Course of Their Self-Neglect

Adina, age 68, whose self-neglect is manifest in hoarding, slovenly appearance, dirty clothes, and unclean and neglected surroundings, described her transition to self-neglect as a crisis stage filled with suffering:

I worked cleaning houses for years . . . and when I was 50, I had a crisis, depression and that, you know, all sorts of things like that and then I asked to be hospitalized . . . that was the outcome of everything I'd seen in my childhood . . . all sorts of things that children shouldn't see . . . I was there about two months and came home . . . I rest, I read, I do crosswords, I try but . . . I cut myself off from my sisters a bit, and I'm sorry about that, and also from my daughter a bit, and from the grandchildren.

Anna, age 68, described her "normal" life and how it changed due to poor health and declining physical capability:

I started suffering from shortness of breath . . . and the house wasn't worth anything in any case. I had plans and all sorts of nice things and carpets and all that, and the cats just about destroyed it all . . . and I want to add another sand box because it smells and the neighbors complained . . . I say I'll do it, but I don't do it, as I haven't the strength . . . my house has turned into a shed . . . this morning, I swept the floor and I wiped over here so that you wouldn't be repulsed . . . and I walk around in the dust and go up to bed and dirty the bed.

Shoshana, age 65, described her reaction to offers of support:

I'm not willing to leave here. They say to me, "You're disabled, you need to live on the ground floor." I said, "I like this place. I like this environment. Why should I move? All my memories are here. . . . The caregiver throws away my newspapers. I got angry with her. She clears me out of everything . . . and she was supposed to help me to shower today, but she was too busy throwing things away . . . if I don't look out for myself, then who will look out for me?"

Martha, age 90, who was aware that others perceived her as "crazy," described her positive traits:

That's my personality, I'm not angry, I don't do anything bad . . . I worked throughout my whole life . . . I always had something else to keep me busy . . . I didn't want another woman to help me . . . I

(continued)

BOX 3.4 Older Adults Describe the Life Course of Their Self-Neglect *(continued)*

know why I don't tell anyone about the way I live; maybe they'll think that I'm a crazy woman . . . thank God I don't have Alzheimer's . . . I'm scared of dying, it's true, I think just like everyone else.

Nehema, age 83, described herself as a compulsive hoarder with an unkempt appearance and living in a filthy environment, but perceived herself as the owner of valuable assets:

I think that every human being has life experience, because everyone has been through something . . . you know already that my soul stays the same even at my age. I'm happy with myself and I know that all beginnings also have an end but I don't think about it. I feel good so I'm happy . . . this is my empire.

Reprinted from Band-Winterstein, Doron, and Naim (2012). Copyright 2012, with permission from Elsevier.

social service or health care professionals approach the topic nonjudgmentally and engage the older adult in problem solving. Similarly, service providers and health care workers may assume that the person does not have the capacity for making appropriate decisions. In these situations, it is imperative to obtain an evaluation of capacity, which is best performed in the context of a comprehensive geriatric assessment. It is also important to consider that services are not being provided because there are no appropriate, acceptable, and affordable ones available. In addition, cultural influences, as discussed in Chapter 5, need to be considered as a factor that can affect both the perception of self-neglect situations and the acceptance of services.

CONSEQUENCES OF SELF-NEGLECT

Although autonomous adults have the right to live in whatever way they choose, self-neglect situations can have serious consequences for the individual, for his or her family and friends, for the surrounding community, for health care providers and services, and sometimes for the welfare of numerous animals. An overriding concern related to consequences is the effect on quality of life for the self-neglecting older adult, which should be the main focus of all involved. This is perhaps the most challenging aspect of self-neglect, as each person involved may define quality of life differently. For self-neglecting older adults, quality of life may depend on preservation of their privacy, independence, and right to choose their living arrangements. For health care providers, quality of life for self-neglecting older adults typically involves minimal standards of personal care and health-related behaviors to prevent serious illness or premature death. For self-neglecters who are animal hoarders, quality of life may be intertwined with relationships with animals; however, the welfare of the animals also needs to be considered.

Data from the Chicago Health and Aging Project cite the following health consequences associated with self-neglect:

- An independent risk factor for death, with a 16-fold increased risk in confirmed severe cases (Dong et al., 2009)
- An independent risk factor for hospitalization (Dong, Simon, & Evans, 2012a)
- Increased 30-day readmissions to hospitals, independent of concomitant medical or social conditions (Dong & Simon, 2015)
- Increased use of hospice and shorter time with hospice before death (Dong & Simon, 2013)
- Substantially higher annual rate of emergency department visits (Dong, Simon, & Evans, 2012b)

Even aside from the consequences on human lives, with the current emphasis on preventable hospitalizations, self-neglect deserves attention as a contributing condition to cost and quality of care.

In addition to being associated with financial consequences for health care systems, self-neglect is associated with consequences for health care providers who are frustrated by their inability to provide effective care. Self-neglect situations often involve ethical dilemmas for nurses, physicians, and other health care providers when they are faced with situations in which legally competent adults engage in behaviors that pose risks to their health. Lastly, home care nurses and other health care providers who perform home visits may be exposed to personal risks when they are required to provide care in an environment that presents risks to health.

Many self-neglecting older adults are socially isolated; however, family and friends who maintain emotional or social connections experience consequences such as distress, frustration, and sadness about the situation. In addition, self-neglect situations involving unsanitary conditions often have consequences for neighbors or apartment residents. For example, infestations of fleas or roaches may affect adjacent apartments and garbage-strewn environments may attract disease-carrying rodents to the neighborhood. Sometimes, these situations involve life-threatening risks for others, as when irresponsible smoking behaviors cause risks for fires.

SELF-NEGLECT AS A CONCERN FOR HEALTH CARE PROVIDERS

For many decades, social service workers and health care providers have addressed self-neglect and hoarding in community-based settings, often in conjunction with adult protective service workers. Physicians, nurses, and other health care professionals have many roles in addressing health-related aspects of self-neglect, as discussed briefly in this section and more comprehensively in Parts II and III of this book. Attention of health care providers is warranted, particularly with regard to management of medical conditions due to nonadherence to recommended treatments. For example, nonadherence with medications is strongly associated with lower functional status and increased risk for self-neglect. One study found that 90% of 100 older adult self-neglecters did not take at least one medication between 80% and 110% of the number of prescribed times, with the mean number of medications that were nonadherent being 3.4 (Turner, Hochschild, Burnett, Zulfiqar, & Dyer, 2012). Although nonadherence with recommended treatments is common among all adults, when noncompliant behaviors cause serious health consequences and there are questions about the person's decision-making capacity, then this may be considered as self-neglect. Another health-related aspect of self-neglect is the common occurrence of nutritional problems, including vitamin deficiencies, malnutrition, and dehydration.

Physicians have addressed medical consequences of self-neglect as a geriatric syndrome. For example, Pavlou and Lachs (2006) reviewed 54 studies and identified the following characteristics indicative of self-neglect as a geriatric syndrome:

- Its multifactorial etiology
- Its clear and independent association with increased mortality
- The fact that two other geriatric syndromes (cognitive impairment and depression) are risk factors for self-neglect

Two years later, these two physicians cited self-neglect as a "growing epidemic" that has profound health and public policy implications for an aging society. They further stated that "physicians of all types will be increasingly called upon to care for these patients, who present a variety of vexing medical, medico-legal, and ethical challenges for which training has not yet prepared them" (Pavlou & Lachs, 2008, p. 1841).

In 2006, three nurses proposed that self-neglect can be designated as a new NANDA nursing diagnosis because self-neglect "presents conceptual, identification, and intervention problems for nurses, health care workers, and for medicolegal systems across settings and in many countries" (Gibbons, Lauder, & Ludwick, 2006, p. 10). The approved NANDA definition of Self-Neglect is "a constellation of culturally framed behaviors involving one or more self-care activities in which there is a failure to maintain a socially accepted standard of health and well-being" (Herdman, 2012, p. 254). Defining characteristics of self-neglect are inadequate personal hygiene, inadequate environmental hygiene, and nonadherence to health activities. In clinical settings, nurses address self-neglect in relation to the following:

- Adherence to prescribed treatment for chronic conditions, such as medication management
- Functional impairments
- Cognitive function and mental health conditions
- Risks for falls and other safety concerns
- Social conditions that create risks, such as lack of appropriate and acceptable support services

Nursing interventions for self-neglecting older adults focus on concomitant conditions, such as functional limitations, self-care deficits, cognitive impairment, and unmanaged or poorly managed medical conditions.

NURSING PERSPECTIVES ON SELF-NEGLECT

Nurses in home care settings address self-neglect not only on a long-term basis but also in the context of the personal environment of the self-neglecting older adult. Interviews with 16 registered nurses providing home care services in a rural area in North Carolina identified several themes related to nursing perceptions of self-neglecting older adults, as summarized in Box 3.5. A dominant theme with particular implications for nursing is that "self-neglect was the 'normal' for these individuals, with clients conducting themselves as if self-neglecting behaviors were ordinary" (Johnson, 2015, p. 34).

BOX 3.5 Home Care Nurses Describe Their Experiences With Clients Who Are Self-Neglecting

Armored: Nurses viewed self-neglecting people as "shielding" themselves as if to protect them from something or someone.

- "It becomes their normal and they just don't see it as being odd or out of the ordinary."
- "They viewed us as an invasion into their homes, their privacy, their independence."
- "When somebody chooses to live off the grid you can't impose what you consider normal on them, because for this that is their normal."

Psychological Derivation: Nurses attributed self-neglect behaviors to psychological reasons, such as dementia, depression, or undiagnosed mental illness.

- "I'm thinking, wow. There's something wrong with someone who doesn't freak out when they see and acknowledge verbally that there are bugs in their wound."
- "There was probably a lot of deep rooted issues that she has never dealt with."

Secluded: Clients were "loners" who either chose to isolate themselves, had families who effectively excommunicated them, or were isolated by circumstances such as death of a spouse.

- "The times I've seen the adult children come to visit it's always with their sense of disgust and they need to get out of there. There's not a good relationship."
- "They shut lots of folks out."
- "There's usually some type of tension between them. Either they don't talk to the adult children, or they visit infrequently."

Nonconformity With Self-Care Conventions: Clients profoundly neglected their personal care or care of their environment.

- "Hair was unkempt, dirty. Nails were outgrown with dirt underneath. Some were broken half off. . . . She had no motivation getting a bath. I could tell by her teeth that she hadn't maintained herself even as far as daily brushing."
- "If they have incontinence episodes, sometimes they don't clean themselves up completely, or sometimes they don't clean themselves up at all."

(continued)

BOX 3.5 Home Care Nurses Describe Their Experiences With Clients Who Are Self-Neglecting *(continued)*

- "One case I can remember in particular, there was just roaches everywhere and the man had had his scalp literally like lifted away. I think the incision was like 32 centimeters long. And then when you peeled the scalp back he had roaches on there. And you know his wife picked up that medicine box and went over there and slammed it on the counter and the roaches went running everywhere . . . I would be flipping out if I saw a roach at my house. But a roach crawling on them is not a big deal."

Adapted from Johnson (2015). Used with permission.

NURSING INTERVENTIONS RELATED TO SELF-NEGLECT

Self-neglect as a unique form of elder abuse is perhaps most pertinent to nursing care across all clinical settings because nurses have numerous opportunities to address contributing factors. Sometimes relatively simple measures, such as connecting a socially isolated older adult to available community resources, can be effective in preventing the development or progression of self-neglect situations. In addition, nurses can use a wide range of nursing skills to address nonadherence to interventions for chronic conditions. Also, nurses have essential roles in addressing executive dysfunction as a common contributing condition in self-neglect situations. For example, nurses can facilitate assessment of cognitive function, assure that treatable causes of cognitive impairment are identified and managed, and assure that interventions are implemented to improve the older adult's cognitive function. Similarly, nurses have essential roles in addressing functional limitations, both directly in care plans and indirectly through referrals for rehabilitation therapists.

Nurses address self-neglect not only through nursing assessments and interventions related to contributing conditions, but also as members of interdisciplinary teams addressing the broader context of each unique self-neglect situation. Finally, in all situations of self-neglect, nurses have opportunities to assure that the rights of the older adult are respected and that the person's capacity is assessed appropriately.

These aspects require sensitivity to cultural values and often involve ethical issues, as discussed in Chapters 5 and 8.

KEY POINTS: WHAT NURSES NEED TO KNOW AND CAN DO

- In the United States, self-neglect is the most frequently encountered form of elder abuse addressed by adult protective service agencies.

- Risks for self-neglect include physical disability or medical conditions, cognitive impairment or mental illness, and inadequate social supports.

- Cognitive characteristics are considered in relation to self-neglecting older adults from two perspectives: as risks for self-neglect, and as a major factor in determining the older adult's capacity for decision making.

- Hoarding and self-neglect typically involve risks to health and safety within the person's environment.

- Self-neglect is a concern for health care providers with respect to individual older adults and the consequences affecting other people and broader environments.

- Nurses have numerous roles in addressing conditions that contribute to self-neglect.

REFERENCES

Aamodt, W. W., Terracina, K. A., & Schillerstrom, J. E. (2015). Cognitive profiles of elder adult protective services clients living in squalor. *Journal of Elder Abuse & Neglect, 27,* 65–73.

Andersen, E., Raffin-Bouchal, S., & Marcy-Edwards, D. (2013). Do they think I am a pack rat? *Journal of Elder Abuse & Neglect, 25,* 438–452.

Band-Winterstein, T., Doron, I., & Naim, S. (2012). Elder self-neglect: A geriatric syndrome or a life course story. *Journal of Aging Studies, 26,* 109–118.

Choi, N. G., Kim, J., & Asseff, J. (2009). Self-neglect and neglect of vulnerable older adults: Reexamination of etiology. *Journal of Gerontological Social Work, 52,* 171–187.

Day, M. R., Leahy-Warren, P., & McCarthy, G. (2013). Perceptions and views of self-neglect: A client-centered perspective. *Journal of Elder Abuse & Neglect, 25,* 76–94.

Dong, X. Q., & Simon, M. (2013). Association between elder self-neglect and hospice utilization in a community population. *Archives of Gerontology and Geriatrics, 56*, 192–198.

Dong, X. Q., & Simon, M. (2015). Elder self-neglect is associated with an increased rate of 30-day hospital readmission: Findings from the Chicago Health and Aging Project. *Gerontology, 61*, 41–50.

Dong, X. Q., Simon, M., & Evans, D. (2012a). Elder self-neglect and hospitalization: Findings from the Chicago Health and Aging Project. *Journal of the American Geriatrics Society, 60*(2), 202–209.

Dong, X. Q., Simon, M., & Evans, D. (2012b). Prospective study of elder self-neglect and ED use in a community population. *American Journal of Emergency Medicine, 30*, 553–561.

Dong, X. Q., Simon, M., Fulmer, T., Mendes de Leon, C., Rajan, B., & Evans, D. A. (2010). Physical function decline and the risk of elder self-neglect in a community-dwelling population. *Gerontologist, 50*, 316–326.

Dong, X. Q., Simon, M., Mendes de Leon, C., Fulmer, T., Beck, T., Hebert, L., ... Evans, D. A. (2009). Elder self-neglect and abuse and mortality risk in a community-dwelling population. *Journal of the American Medical Association, 302*(5), 517–526.

Dyer, C., Goodwin, J., Pickens-Pace, S., Burnett, J., & Kelly, P. A. (2007). Self-neglect among the elderly: A model based on more than 500 patients seen by a geriatric medicine team. *American Journal of Public Health, 97*, 1671–1676.

Ernst, J. S., & Smith, C. A. (2011). Adult protective services clients confirmed for self-neglect: Characteristics and service use. *Journal of Elder Abuse & Neglect, 23*, 289–303.

Frost, R. O., Patronek, G., & Rosenfield, E. (2011). A comparison of object and animal hoarding. *Depression and Anxiety, 28*, 885–891.

Gibbons, S., Lauder, W., & Ludwick, R. (2006). Self-neglect: A proposed new NANDA diagnosis. *International Journal of Nursing Terminology and Classification, 17*, 10–18.

Gruenberg, E. M., Brandon, S., & Kasius, R. V. (1966). Identifying cases of social breakdown syndrome. *Millbank Memorial Fund Quarterly, 44*(Suppl.), 150–155.

Herdman, T. H. (Ed.). (2012). *NANDA International Nursing Diagnoses: Definitions & classification, 2012–2014*. Oxford, UK: Wiley-Blackwell.

Iris, M., Conrad, K. J., & Ridings, J. (2014). Observational measure of self-neglect. *Journal of Elder Abuse & Neglect, 26*, 365–397.

Johnson, Y. O. (2015). Home care nurses' experiences with and perceptions of elder self-neglect. *Home Healthcare Now, 33*, 31–37.

Macmillan, D., & Shaw, P. (1966). Senile breakdown in standards of personal and environmental cleanliness. *British Medical Journal, 2*, 1032–1037.

Nathanson, J. N. (2009). Animal hoarding: Slipping into the darkness of comorbid animal and self-neglect. *Journal of Elder Abuse & Neglect, 21*, 307–324.

National Adult Protective Services Association. (n.d.). *Get informed: Other safety concerns and self-neglect.* Retrieved from www.napsa-now.org

Patronek, G. J. (1999). Hoarding of animals: An under-recognized public health problem in a difficult-to-study population. *Public Health Reports, 114,* 81–87.

Pavlou, M. P., & Lachs, M. (2006). Could self-neglect in older adults be a geriatric syndrome? *Journal of the American Geriatrics Society, 54,* 831–842.

Pavlou, M. P., & Lachs, M. (2008). Self-neglect in older adults: A primer for clinicians. *Journal of General Internal Medicine, 23,* 1841–1846.

Reyes-Ortiz, C. A., Burnett, J., Flores, D. V., Halphen, J. M., & Dyer, C. B. (2014). Medical implications of elder abuse: Self-neglect. *Clinics in Geriatric Medicine, 30,* 807–823.

Schillerstrom, J. E., Birkenfeld, E. M., Yu, A. S., Le, M. P. T., Goldstein, D. J., & Royall, D. R. (2013). Neuropsychological correlates of performance based functional status in elder adult protective services (APS) referrals for capacity assessment. *Journal of Elder Abuse & Neglect, 25,* 294–304.

Taylor, B. J., Killick, C., O'Brien, M., Begley, E., & Carter-Anand, J. (2014). Older people's conceptualization of elder abuse and neglect. *Journal of Elder Abuse & Neglect, 26,* 223–243.

Turner, A., Hochschild, A., Burnett, J., Zulfiqar, A., & Dyer, C. B. (2012). High prevalence of medication non-adherence in a sample of community-dwelling older adults with adult protective services-validated self neglect. *Drugs & Aging, 29,* 741–749.

ELDER ABUSE IN LONG-TERM CARE FACILITIES

The topic of elder abuse in long-term care settings is relevant not only to nurses who work in these facilities, but also to nurses in any setting where residents of long-term care facilities receive acute or intermittent care. This chapter presents an overview of different types of long-term care facilities, describes forms of elder abuse that occur in these facilities, and provides information about resources for addressing elder abuse. In addition, the topic of nursing responsibilities with regard to elder abuse when it occurs in long-term care settings is addressed in the last section and illustrated in several case examples.

OVERVIEW: LONG-TERM CARE FACILITIES

The term *long-term care facilities* refers to a wide range of settings, including nursing homes (also called nursing facilities or skilled care facilities), assisted living facilities, and board and care homes. Definitions and descriptions vary significantly and are influenced not only by all levels of governmental agencies but also by each institution and by public perception. There is no universal definition of these settings, but they can be broadly categorized as either nursing homes or residential care facilities. Certain characteristics are associated with each of these broad categories, as delineated in Table 4.1 and described in the following sections.

TABLE 4.1 Differences Between Nursing Homes and Residential Care Facilities

CHARACTERISTICS	NURSING HOMES	RESIDENTIAL CARE FACILITIES
Source of funds	Medicare, Medicaid, Veterans Administration, other health care insurance, self-pay, private long-term care insurance	Primarily self-pay (including some payments from private long-term care policies); under certain circumstances, payments are available through Medicaid, the Veterans Administration, or other federal programs
Licensure and inspections	Federal Medicare and Medicaid guidelines, state regulatory agencies, strict standards of care	States establish requirements for licensure and regulation of various types of residential care facilities, and these vary widely; some residential care facilities are not covered by state laws because of small size; the small percentage of facilities that receive federal funds comply with federal regulations
Philosophical orientation	Based primarily on medical models, with emphasis on person-centered care to address complex health-related needs of residents	Based primarily on social nonmedical models, with medical services provided secondarily (often by outside service providers)
Skill level of workers	Federal laws delineate minimal staffing levels and requirements for licensed health care professionals	Because services are designated as "nonmedical," there are no federal requirements for licensed health care professionals; state laws vary widely and do not necessarily include requirements for licensed health care professionals

Care in Nursing Homes

Nursing homes are held to clearly defined standards of care because facilities that receive Medicare and Medicaid funds have been subject to federal regulations for decades. However, it is important to recognize that as of 2016, these federal regulations did not clearly define elder abuse in nursing homes. Moreover, there is some variation in the way state agencies enforce these regulations. State agencies inspect nursing homes regularly to identify deficiencies, with much attention to quality of care provided for residents. Information about deficiencies and corrective actions is available in readily accessible government reports and websites. Deficiencies that cause harm or immediate jeopardy to residents are particularly relevant to elder abuse. Data indicate that in 2014, more than one in five facilities received a deficiency for actual harm or jeopardy (Harrington, Carrillo, & Garfield, 2015).

Care in Residential Care Facilities

Residential care facilities include assisted living facilities, board and care homes, and any type of group setting that provides care for adults with varying degrees of dependency or types of impairments. These facilities are licensed and regulated at the state level, and all states have at least one category of residential care. In 2014, the Centers for Medicare & Medicaid Services established minimum requirements for those residential care facilities that receive Medicaid funds for services. Residents of Medicaid-funded facilities include adults with disabilities, such as chronic mental illness or developmental disabilities, and older adults who have a low income and would otherwise need care in a nursing home.

States and geographic regions vary widely with regard to the following aspects of residential care facilities: (a) definitions, (b) types available, (c) staffing requirements, (d) services provided, (e) procedures for enforcing regulations, and (f) extent of public funding. Descriptions of these facilities typically include phrases such as "independent with care" or "supportive care," but responsibilities of the staff or the institution are not always well defined. In general, care in residential care facilities is defined as "nonmedical" and includes personal care assistance, transportation, and social and recreational opportunities. When lines of responsibilities are vague, as they often are in residential care facilities, it is difficult to determine whether the staff are responsible for neglect or whether the resident is self-neglecting. Another source of concern is that residents of these facilities can socially isolate themselves; this is a risk factor for elder abuse occurring and being undetected.

A trend in health care services that is of growing concern is the increasing rate of admission to residential care facilities for older adults who have complicated and unstable mental and physical health problems (Phillips, Guo, & Kim, 2013). Concerns also arise when the needs of residents change significantly after they are admitted and all parties involved (i.e., the resident, the family, the facility, and others involved with decision making) resist a plan that requires a move, even though the care provided no longer meets the resident's health-related needs. A concern pertinent to elder abuse is that residential care facilities are developing at a rapid pace, with many variations in the services provided, and there is significant lag time on both the federal and state levels before laws and regulations are developed. Thus, quality of care varies widely and less information is available about the care provided or the occurrence of elder abuse in residential care facilities.

ELDER ABUSE IN LONG-TERM CARE FACILITIES

Although discussions of elder abuse in long-term care settings typically focus on neglectful or abusive actions of nursing assistants and other direct care staff, in reality, it occurs in all forms and arises from many sources. Sources include administrators, direct care workers, families, friends, visitors, and other residents. A broad definition of resident abuse that emerged through data analysis and interviews with 10 registered nurses working in long-term care facilities is that abuse occurred when the resident perceived hurt, whether or not the hurt was intentional (Hirst, 2002). This chapter discusses causes of and risk factors for elder abuse in long-term care facilities and focuses on types that are most directly within the scope of nursing responsibilities. Financial exploitation and sexual abuse of long-term residents as aspects of elder abuse are addressed in Chapters 15 and 16.

Causes and Risk Factors

Administrators, including nursing supervisors, are accountable for allowing an institutional environment that creates risks for elder abuse by direct care workers. For example, high workload, inadequate staff training, and staff burnout are conditions that are strongly associated with elder abuse in long-term care facilities. Other conditions that foster an environment of elder abuse in long-term care facilities are high staff turnover, lack of support and recognition, lack of policies and procedures for care, poor screening of personnel prior to employment, and lack of supervision and periodic evaluations.

Numerous reports since the 1990s have documented a significant and positive relationship between nurse staffing levels and quality of care in nursing homes (Harrington et al., 2015). There is widespread agreement that two major interventions for preventing elder abuse in long-term care facilities are increased staffing of nursing and other direct care workers and improved staff education related to care of residents (Hirschel & Anetzberger, 2012).

Individual staff characteristics associated with increased risk of mistreating a resident are personal stresses and negative attitudes toward residents. In addition, lack of understanding of resident behaviors, particularly dementia-related behaviors, is a major risk for mistreatment of long-term care residents. For example, staff may view their own abusive actions as justifiable responses in retaliation to aggressive behaviors of residents.

Characteristics of Residents

Dementia and dependency on others for care, which are often characteristics of long-term care residents, are characteristics that increase the risk for elder abuse. The risk is heightened when the person also exhibits dementia-related behaviors that the caregiver finds difficult or disturbing (e.g., aggressive or combative behaviors). National data indicate that 46% of nursing home residents had a dementia diagnosis in 2014 and 31% had psychiatric conditions such as schizophrenia or mood disorders (Harrington et al., 2015). Although dementia is associated with increased risk for all forms of elder abuse, resident-to-resident aggression is a type that is strongly associated with dementia-related behaviors and is being addressed in long-term care settings, as discussed later in this chapter.

ELDER ABUSE BY DIRECT CARE STAFF

The most obvious cases of elder abuse by direct care staff workers are associated with verbal or physical mistreatment and inadequate care (i.e., neglect). Staff actions or omissions, which may be intentional or unintentional, are considered abusive when they harm the resident. Acts of omission, such as not answering call lights in a timely manner, or acts of commission, such as verbal abuse, may or may not cause immediate physical harm, but they can cause immediate and long-term emotional harm. Examples of elder abuse by direct care staff in nursing homes include the following:

- Excessive use of physical or chemical restraints
- Lack of adequate time for activities of daily living
- Not allowing residents to perform self-care tasks that they are capable of doing
- Lack of oral care
- Delays in answering call lights
- Removing or turning off call lights
- Lack of ambulation
- Expression of anger toward a resident
- Disrespectful or infantilizing tone of voice or choice of words
- Unnecessary or unwanted touching, especially around breasts or genitalia
- Invasive procedures, such as rectal examinations, that are unnecessary for patient care

Residents may perceive some actions that are unintentional, or even well-intentioned, on the part of direct care staff as abusive or neglectful. For example, residents of long-term care facilities commonly complain that they feel rushed and are not allowed to perform self-care tasks, whereas direct-care staff feel they are doing the best they can within the limits of their time.

"OK, that's enough grandma, shut up!" We see this type of thing regularly. Or "Come on, granny, let's go wash your behind!" That's no way to speak to an 80-year-old woman! (Charpentier & Soulieres, 2013, p. 347)

Two issues related to elder abuse that are directly within the responsibility of licensed nurses in long-term care facilities are misuse of psychotropic medications and the use of physical restraints. The federal government has been addressing these issues in nursing homes since the late 1980s, and some progress has been made; however, 26% of nursing home citations were related to the inappropriate use of psychotropic medications in 2014 (Harrington et al., 2015). Medication mismanagement has also been identified as an aspect of elder abuse in residential care facilities and includes nursing staff denying access to medication, giving excessive medication, or inappropriately delaying the administration of medications (Castle, Ferguson-Rome, & Teresi, 2015).

There is a great deal of controversy about medication management in residential care facilities because some state laws permit unlicensed personnel to administer medications, although usually with some restrictions. In particular, serious questions have been raised about allowing unlicensed staff to administer as needed psychotropic medications for behavioral conditions (Carder, O'Keefe, & O'Keefe, 2015). These controversies make it difficult to identify lines of responsibility related to misuse of psychotropic medications and overall mismanagement of medications.

Aspects of elder abuse in long-term care settings that are often unrecognized by staff are (a) the imposition of unwanted or unnecessary care that diminishes the resident's self-esteem as well as his or her ability to maintain independence and (b) psychological abuse that is often experienced by nursing home residents as an unintentional consequence of circumstances inherent in the setting. For example, even though nursing homes are viewed as "homes," administrators and staff exert considerable control over the care, services, and schedules provided to all residents. Long-term care facilities vary widely in the degree of person-centered care they provide, but even in the best facilities, residents experience an unbalance of power by virtue of depending on others for daily care. One elder abuse scholar noted that in the nursing home context, abuse such as insulting remarks may be extremely important given the circumscribed locus of control that exists for many residents. When impaired residents have few interactions with friends, family, or others, interactions with nursing home staff caregivers may be the most important interactions of their daily lives. In this context, no cases of elder abuse from staff caregivers can be considered benign (Castle, 2012).

RESIDENT-TO-RESIDENT AGGRESSION

Resident-to-resident aggression (also called resident-to-resident abuse, violence, or mistreatment) is considered a unique type of elder abuse that occurs in all types of long-term care settings. Resident-to-resident aggression is defined as "negative, aggressive and intrusive verbal, physical, sexual, and material interactions between long-term care residents that in a community setting would likely be unwelcome and potentially cause physical or psychological distress or harm to the recipient"

(McDonald et al., 2015). This definition encompasses a broad range of experiences ranging from the imposition of unwanted assistance to serious physical injury, sexual abuse, or even death at the most serious end. Pillemer and colleagues (2011) analyzed 139 events of resident-to-resident aggression and categorized these incidents as follows:

■ Invasion of privacy or personal integrity (e.g., inappropriate caregiving, verbal or physical threats)

■ Roommate problems (e.g., belligerent, repetitious, or antagonistic behaviors)

■ Hostile interpersonal interaction (e.g., angry or controlling statements, sarcasm, accusations)

■ Unprovoked aggressive actions

■ Inappropriate sexual behavior (e.g., unwanted advances, intentional exposure)

Box 4.1 provides an overview of strategies for managing resident-to-resident abuse, based on an evidence-based model called the SEARCH approach.

The experience of "bullying" has been addressed as an aspect of resident-to-resident aggression. This concept is typically associated with an imbalance of power, which can be very subtle among residents of long-term care facilities. It is not uncommon for residents who have a limitation in one aspect of functioning (e.g., memory loss) to talk loudly in a demeaning manner to someone with another type of disability (e.g., mobility impairment). This is often evident in group dining room settings when a resident refuses to sit with certain other residents. Although the rights of individual residents need to be respected, staff also need to take action when this type of resident-to-resident interaction is detrimental to one of the residents.

> There's one woman here who is really impossible to live with. She has no respect for anyone. She has a motorized chair and runs into everyone in the elevator. No one says or does anything . . . I've seen 3 or 4 incidents, and she's going to end up injuring someone. (Charpentier & Soulieres, 2013, p. 348)

ADDRESSING ELDER ABUSE THAT OCCURS IN LONG-TERM CARE FACILITIES

Elder abuse that occurs in long-term care facilities is being addressed at many levels as a major focus of quality of care. The Centers for

BOX 4.1 Strategies for Managing Resident-to-Resident Abuse

Support

- Attend to injuries
- Listen to all residents involved
- Validate residents' fears and frustrations

Evaluate

- Identify needed actions
- Evaluate all residents involved, including those who witnessed the event

Act

- Attend to the needs of all the residents involved
- Separate the residents
- Acknowledge grievances and concerns of all residents

Report

- Report to nursing supervisor and all appropriate authorities or agencies
- Contact families if appropriate
- Document the event in residents' charts

Care Plan

- Update care plans for all residents involved
- Talk with care team to identify ways of intervening and avoiding episodes
- Assess and document residents' preferences for privacy and routines
- Obtain appropriate medical and psychiatric evaluations

Help Avoid

- Avoid overcrowding of residents
- Recognize and address risk factors
- Separate residents known to have negative interactions

Adapted from Ellis et al. (2014).

Medicare & Medicaid Services and the Elder Justice Act currently support national initiatives to improve care in facilities that receive federal funds. States are also addressing many issues related to care in residential care facilities, but these efforts vary widely. In many areas of the country, the development of newer models of long-term care has led to competition to attract residents; in turn, this has led to a focus on person-centered care.

Long-Term Care Ombudsman Programs

Major concerns about quality of care in nursing homes that began during the 1960s led to the establishment of the Nursing Home Ombudsman program in 1972. This program has gradually expanded—as reflected in changing the name to the Long-Term Care Ombudsman program in 1981—and it has become a major resource for addressing issues related to care in all nursing homes and residential care facilities. Today, Long-Term Care Ombudsman programs are available in every state, the District of Columbia, Guam, and Puerto Rico, as a major resource for investigation and resolution of any aspect of care in long-term care facilities.

The federal government provides funds and establishes regulations for all Long-Term Care Ombudsman programs, but the programs are administered at state levels. Most states also have local offices. A major mandate of all State Long-Term Care Ombudsman programs is to "identify, investigate, and resolve complaints that (1) are made by or on behalf of residents; and (2) relate to actions, inactions, or decisions, that may adversely affect the health, safety, welfare and rights of residents" (Federal Register, 2015, p. 7761). Long-Term Care Ombudsman programs investigate complaints only after receiving consent from the resident or someone legally acting on behalf of the resident. This characteristic distinguishes the approach of the Long-Term Care Ombudsman from that of adult protective services, which does not require the consent of the older adult to initiate an investigation. Another distinguishing feature is the broad scope of ombudsman programs with regard to types of complaints that they investigate. About 30% of complaints are related to care, or lack of care, and the ombudsman programs are "on the front line in identifying abuse" (Miller, 2012).

Depending on the state, when a situation of elder abuse is suspected, Long-Term Care Ombudsman programs may investigate, refer the case to local adult protective services or designated agencies, or jointly investigate the complaint with other agencies. In recent years, some state and local ombudsman programs have been designated as the lead agency for receiving and investigating reports of abuse in all long-term care facilities (Hollister & Estes, 2012). When an abuse report is substantiated, further investigation is carried out by the state agency responsible for licensure and certification of the facility, and also by the state professional licensing authority when the abuse is committed by a professional.

Responsibilities of Nurses in All Health Care Settings

Nurses may find evidence of elder abuse when residents of long-term care facilities receive care in hospitals, emergency departments, or outpatient settings. For example, conditions such as bruises, dehydration, malnutrition, and pressure ulcers can be indicators of neglect or other types of elder abuse. Nurses who work in hospice or home care agencies may observe neglectful or abusive situations when they provide care for residents of long-term care facilities. Nurses in all health care settings are required to report suspected cases of elder abuse for investigation, as discussed in Chapter 6.

Situations involving neglect or poor care of long-term care residents that are not at the level of abuse can be addressed by Long-Term Care Ombudsman programs. Nurses can call the local Long-Term Care Ombudsman program to discuss situations when they have concerns about the care of a resident. These programs work toward resolution of a broad range of complaints and serve an advocacy role for residents of all long-term care facilities. In addition, nurses in all settings have opportunities to teach older adults or their concerned family members about the services of Long-Term Care Ombudsman programs and provide information about the local office. Appendix B lists websites and contact information for all Long-Term Care Ombudsman program state offices.

Responsibilities of Nurses Who Work in Long-Term Care Facilities

In addition to state laws related to reporting suspected cases of elder abuse, the 2010 Elder Justice Act is a federal law that specifically requires nurses who work in long-term care facilities and contract agencies (e.g., hospice, advanced practice nurses) to immediately report suspected abuse to both the appropriate local authorities (e.g., adult protective services, law enforcement agencies) and to the state survey agency. Additional provisions of this act related to reporting abuse in long-term care facilities are as follows: (a) An employee who files a complaint is protected from any form of retribution, and (b) individuals who fail to report can be fined and will no longer be able to work in any federally funded program.

Although reporting suspected cases meets legal responsibilities, it does not address the numerous opportunities nurses have to prevent the onset or escalation of elder abuse in long-term care facilities. An important, and relatively easy-to-implement, intervention is to make a conscious effort to demonstrate respect for each individual resident through verbal and nonverbal interactions, with particular attention to actions and verbalizations that a resident might interpret as disrespectful. This intervention is effective not only for providing good care but also for role modeling for staff and others who interact with residents.

Licensed nursing staff in long-term care facilities usually have a combination of administrative or supervisory responsibilities and direct care activities. In these roles, nurses can address elder abuse in the following ways:

- Use appropriate interventions to address dementia-associated behaviors and avoid using psychotropic medications.

- Support restraint-free care.

- Assure that direct care staff are respectful in verbal and nonverbal interactions with residents.

- Listen to residents to gain insight on their perspectives about the care they receive.

- Assure that care plans address needs of residents while at the same time allowing and encouraging self-care within the abilities and wishes of each resident.

- Advocate for appropriate staffing levels.

- Advocate for staff training, particularly with regard to effective management of behavioral manifestations of dementia.

- Advocate for policies that support person-centered care.

The following case examples describe interventions that nurses in all settings can use to address elder abuse when it occurs in long-term care facilities.

CASE EXAMPLES OF WHAT NURSES CAN DO TO ADDRESS ELDER ABUSE WHEN IT OCCURS IN LONG-TERM CARE FACILITIES

CASE 4.1 When Unnecessary Care Is Provided

Clinical Situation: Mrs. Rothermel at Sunnydale Nursing Home

Mrs. Rothermel is an 81-year-old resident of Sunnydale Nursing Home who was admitted after surgery for a hip fracture. She had been independent in her own home until she fell and fractured her hip while walking to the mailbox 16 months ago. Although she progressed in rehabilitation, she has remained in the nursing home because she requires supervision with activities of daily living due to cognitive impairments. In addition, she has been admitted to the hospital twice during the past year for heart failure and is unable to manage her medications. The physical therapist states she is able to walk with a walker and "standby assistance," but nursing staff regularly use a wheelchair whenever she is out of her room.

What Nurse Yolanda Does

When Nurse Yolanda is administering medications to Mrs. Rothermel, she asks if the resident will be attending the afternoon social activity. Mrs. Rothermel says, "I've stopped going to those activities because I don't like to be wheeled around in one of those clunky chairs. If I stay in my room, I'm free to walk around by myself, but the aides insist on putting me in a wheelchair whenever I want to leave my room. They say they are worried that I'll fall, but I think it's because they are lazy and they think I'm an imbecile. If I have to keep living here like that, I will become useless."

Nurse Yolanda reviews the notes from the recent plan of care meeting and confirms that Mrs. Rothermel is safe to walk with her walker with standby assistance. She talks with nursing assistants and adds a notation to the daily care plan that nursing staff should provide standby assistance with walking at least once every shift. In addition, she talks with Mrs. Rothermel about the plan and returns the wheelchair to the storage area.

CASE 4.2 When a Long-Term Care Resident Has Been Neglected

Clinical Situation: Mr. Blackburn, Resident of a Dementia Assisted Living Facility

Mr. Blackburn, who is 87 years old, was brought to the emergency department by his daughter, Sonia, for evaluation of a change in his mental status. Sonia reports that he has resided in a dementia assisted living facility for 6 months and needed only a minimal level of care when he was admitted. Sonia lives out of town and had not visited in 3 months, but she maintained phone contact with the assistant director of the facility, who always assured her that her father was "doing well." When Sonia visited earlier today, she was concerned about the major decline in his cognition as well as his physical appearance. He had lost weight, was unshaven, and had a strong body odor. Moreover, she could not find his eyeglasses, hearing aids, or dentures in his room. He did not recognize Sonia and talked "nonsensically" about animals in cages as he pointed out the window. When Sonia asked the assistant director about the changes, she was told "You know, your father has dementia, and these changes are bound to happen. He gets upset when we try to help him, so we allow him to be independent." Sonia was able to help her father to her car so she could bring him to the emergency department.

What Nurse Martin Does

Nurse Martin assesses Mr. Blackburn in the emergency department and documents the following abnormal findings:

Vital signs: T 100.1° oral, P 98, slightly irregular, R 24, BP 168/70

Skin: dry, pale, turgor poor over chest, stage 2 pressure ulcer (round, 3-cm diameter) over coccyx, both heels reddened

Mouth/lips: oral mucous membrane dry, tongue red, cracks at sides of lips

Mental status: alert, oriented to own name, calls his daughter by the name of his deceased wife, states he is in prison cell

Sensory: unable to hear ticking watch when held close to either ear, no hearing aids available, understands loud voices

(continued)

CASE 4.2 When a Long-Term Care Resident Has Been Neglected *(continued)*

Nurse Martin also documents a summary of the concerns and information that Sonia has reported.

After several hours in the emergency department, Mr. Blackburn is admitted to the geriatric assessment unit with the following medical diagnoses: acute change in mental status, urinary tract infection, stage 2 pressure ulcer, and dehydration. When Sonia asks Nurse Martin's advice about a plan for her father, he tells her that the geriatric assessment team will recommend a suitable level of long-term care after his acute problems are resolved and he has reached his best level of functioning. In addition, Nurse Martin tells Sonia that she can meet with the social worker in the geriatric assessment unit within the next couple of days and she can also call the Long-Term Care Ombudsman for information about long-term care facilities that she can begin to look at. He also reports the case for investigation to the local adult protective services office, and informs Sonia about the report.

CASE 4.3 When Medications Are Not Being Administered Properly

Clinical Situation: Betty Andrews at Hillsview Assisted Living

Betty Andrews is 89 years old and moved to Hillsview Assisted Living 5 years ago because her mobility was limited due to osteoarthritis in her knees, hips, and spine. Although Betty used a wheelchair most of the time, she enjoyed social activities in the facility and trips in the van with other residents. Her care plan included 1-hour daily assistance with personal care and transferring. Her medications were kept in a locked drawer in her room, and staff provided access to her medications so she could self-administer them twice daily. Betty's quality of life at Hillsview was good until 8 months ago when she was diagnosed with lung cancer. She has become increasingly dependent in her daily care needs, and Betty's family has supplemented the care

(continued)

CASE 4.3 When Medications Are Not Being Administered Properly *(continued)*

provided by Hillsview with personal care aides from Hillsview Comfort Care. One month ago, Betty began experiencing severe pain and a referral was made to hospice.

Nurse Andrea, Hillsview Community Hospice and Palliative Care Association

During Nurse Andrea's initial assessment, she finds that Betty is quite anxious and uncomfortable. Betty describes her pain level as "usually 7 on a scale of 1 to 10 and sometimes up to 9." The aide from Comfort Care reports that Betty sleeps only for short periods and constantly complains of pain. When Nurse Andrea asks about the administration of medications, she is told that Betty takes her medications twice daily when the medication drawer is unlocked. Although there are physician orders for as-needed medications for anxiety and pain, Betty has not received any because neither the staff at the assisted living facility nor the aides from Comfort Care are permitted to administer medications. Nurse Andrea addresses the situation by talking with the administrator of the facility and Betty and her family to request that Betty's level of care be increased to include administration of medications by the licensed practical nurse, who is available at all times. Betty and her family are agreeable to paying for the higher level of care, and Nurse Andrea is able to work with the licensed practical nurse at Hillsview to improve symptom management for Betty.

KEY POINTS: WHAT NURSES NEED TO KNOW AND CAN DO

- Within the categories of nursing homes and residential care facilities, facilities differ significantly in the level of care provided and regulations related to care.

- Residents of long-term care facilities can experience all forms of elder abuse.

- Sources of elder abuse in long-term care facilities include staff, visitors, and other residents.

■ The Long-Term Care Ombudsman program is a major resource in all parts of the United States for addressing concerns about quality of care, including elder abuse and neglect, for residents of nursing homes and residential care facilities.

■ Nurses in all health care settings can observe for situations of neglect or abuse and report suspected cases to adult protective services.

■ It is important to teach older adults and families to use the Long-Term Care Ombudsman program as a resource for addressing concerns about care provided to any resident of a long-term care facility.

■ Nurses who work in long-term care settings can implement the following interventions to prevent and address elder abuse: role model and teach respectful interactions with all residents, avoid unnecessary administration of psychotropic medications, use the interventions in Box 4.1 for resident-to-resident abuse, and develop and implement person-centered care plans.

REFERENCES

Carder, P., O'Keefe, J., & O'Keefe, C. (2015, June 15). *Compendium of residential care and assisted living regulations and policy: 2015 edition.* Washington, DC: U.S. Department of Health and Human Services.

Castle, N. (2012). Nurse aides' reports of resident abuse in nursing homes. *Journal of Applied Gerontology, 31,* 402–422.

Castle, N., Ferguson-Rome, J. C., & Teresi, J. A. (2015). Elder abuse in residential long-term care: An update to the 2003 National Research Council Report. *Journal of Applied Gerontology, 34,* 2407–2443.

Charpentier, M., & Soulieres, M. (2013). Elder abuse and neglect in institutional settings: The resident's perspective. *Journal of Elder Abuse & Neglect, 25,* 330–354.

Ellis, J., Teresi, J., Ramirez, M., Silver, S., Boratgis, G., Kong J., . . . Pillemer, K. A. (2014). Managing resident to resident elder mistreatment (R-REM) in nursing homes: The SEARCH approach. *Journal of Continuing Education in Nursing, 45*(3), 112–123.

Federal Register. (2015, February 11). *Rules and Regulations, Part 1327— Allotments for vulnerable elder rights protection activities.* Washington, DC: U.S. Department of Health and Human Services.

Harrington, C., Carrillo, H., & Garfield, R. (2015). *Nursing facilities, staffing, residents and facility deficiencies, 2009 through 2014.* The Kaiser Commission on Medicaid and the uninsured. Retrieved from kkf.org.

Hirschel, A. E., & Anetzberger, G. J. (2012). Evaluating and enhancing federal responses to abuse and neglect in long-term care facilities. *Public Policy & Aging Report, 22*(1), 22–27.

Hirst, S. P. (2002). Defining resident abuse within the culture of long-term care institutions. *Clinical Nursing Research, 11,* 267–283.

Hollister, B. A., & Estes, C. (2012). Local Long-Term Care Ombudsman program effectiveness and the measurement of program resources. *Journal of Applied Gerontology, 32,* 708–728.

McDonald, L., Hitzig, M., Pillemer, K., Lachs, M., Beaulieu, M., Brownell, P., . . . Thomas, C. (2015). Developing a research agenda on resident-to-resident aggression: Recommendations from a consensus conference. *Journal of Elder Abuse & Neglect, 27,* 146–167.

Miller, M. (2012). Ombudsman on the front line: Improving quality of care and preventing abuse in nursing homes. *Generations, 36*(3), 60–63.

Phillips, L. R., Guo, G., & Kim, H. (2013). Elder mistreatment in U. S. residential care facilities: The scope of the problem. *Journal of Elder Abuse & Neglect, 25,* 19–39.

Pillemer, K., Chen, E. K., Van Haitsma, K., Teresi, J., Ramirez, M., Silver, S., . . . Lachs, M. S. (2011). Resident-to-resident aggression in nursing homes: Results from a qualitative event reconstruction study. *Gerontologist, 52,* 24–43.

5

CULTURAL CONSIDERATIONS RELATED TO ELDER ABUSE

In the broadest—and most accurate—scope, the topic of cultural considerations related to elder abuse encompasses the wide range of current and past conditions in older adults, perpetrators, and the immediate and broader environments that influence all aspects of defining, reporting, and addressing elder abuse. This scope is not only unwieldy to discuss in a chapter, but is also impossible to cover based on the limited state of research on this topic and the lack of universally accepted definitions of elder abuse. Consistent with the purpose of this book, this chapter presents information about cultural dimensions of elder abuse that are pertinent to nurses caring for older adults who are in situations of actual or potential elder abuse.

This chapter focuses on cultural dimensions in the context of common themes identified by elder abuse scholars and national organizations that are pertinent to elder abuse in diverse populations in the United States. Information is presented about cultural considerations related to elder abuse in the four minority groups designated by the federal government; however, it is imperative to avoid stereotypes and recognize the limitations of current knowledge (as discussed in the next section). Another important point is that these four ethnic groups are heterogeneous and each individual's cultural identity exists on a spectrum and is formed by many factors. In addition, it is imperative to recognize that cultural considerations apply to many groups and subgroups, but information about subgroups and smaller groups (e.g., rural older adults and lesbian, gay, bisexual, and transgender older adults) is very limited and just beginning to emerge.

An underlying premise of this chapter is that nurses are not expected to be experts on all aspects of cultural diversity; however, they are expected to provide care that is culturally appropriate for groups of people for whom they care. They are also expected to be nonjudgmental and avoid stereotypes and identify the unique cultural perspective of individual older adults and families. To achieve this, perhaps the most important part of this chapter is Box 5.1, which can serve as a guide to developing cultural sensitivity about the multiple dimensions of elder abuse.

CULTURAL DIMENSIONS OF ELDER ABUSE

Although it is imperative to avoid generalizations related to any topic, this is especially important with regard to cultural dimensions of elder abuse because of limitations in the current base of knowledge. A few studies related to elder abuse in culturally diverse groups in the United States were published in the 1980s; however, it was not until the late 1990s that national attention was brought to this topic. Studies to date have focused primarily on its prevalence in different groups, but this information is clouded and problematic because there is no single definition of elder abuse and perceptions of abuse are strongly influenced by many factors, including cultural perspectives of all involved.

Additional complicating factors related to information about cultural dimensions of elder abuse are as follows: (a) Information from studies that address one subgroup of a larger ethnic/racial group cannot be generalized to the larger group, and (b) because the number of studies related to elder abuse in a specific group varies widely, the information in this chapter may disproportionately focus on those groups that have been most frequently included in research. Perhaps the most important consideration is that information about cultural influences reflects general characteristics of particular groups, but this information cannot describe characteristics of any individual member of the group. In addition, each individual is influenced by a combination of cultural factors from many sources.

Cultural Influences on Perceptions of Elder Abuse

Although the most blatant situations can readily be defined as abusive, many—if not most—situations encountered in clinical settings are less clearly defined and can be influenced by many factors. As one elder abuse scholar stated, "Mistreatment is, in fact, a culturally relative issue in the sense that cultural groups have their own notions of 'right' and 'wrong' treatment of elders . . .," and what appears to be abusive to the majority may not be interpreted that way by minority groups, who may have unique ways of describing or categorizing abuse (Jervis, 2014, p. 76).

Elder abuse scholars currently emphasize the importance of considering contextual factors that influence perceptions of elder abuse, such as in the following examples:

- Definitions of spousal abuse are strongly influenced by cultural perceptions of men and women.

- Behaviors that go against personal religious beliefs may be perceived as abusive (e.g., if a Hindu older adult lives with children who do not observe the same dietary restrictions, this may be perceived as psychological abuse).

- Definition of financial abuse can vary significantly according to cultural expectations related to intergenerational financial support.

- People with dementia may be viewed as not feeling the effects of abuse.

- People with dementia-related behaviors may be viewed as "deserving" of behaviors that otherwise would be viewed as abusive.

- Actions of a family caregiver who is stressed and well-intentioned may be viewed as less abusive than those of a paid caregiver.

- Acts that do not cause immediate physical consequences may not be perceived as abusive (e.g., ignoring an older adult's request for assistance with toileting may be viewed as acceptable if the person then urinates on a disposable pad).

- Acts that are viewed as protective of the older adult may be considered acceptable (e.g., using restraints to prevent wandering).

Perspective of Korean immigrants who went through the Korean War: Since physical assault doesn't seem as tragic or difficult as what they had to go through before, they don't think of it as something so severe or abusive. (Lee, Kaplan, & Perez-Stable, 2014, p. 12)

In addition, cultural variations in perceptions of autonomy and decision making (as discussed in Chapter 8) can have an effect on legal and ethical aspects of elder abuse and neglect. Cultural influences related to perception of elder abuse by specific groups are discussed in the last sections of this chapter.

Avoidance of Stereotypes Related to Elder Abuse

Avoidance of stereotypes is an important consideration with regard to all aspects of elder abuse, but this is especially important in relation to identification of risk factors. Public and professional publications describing risk factors are useful for identifying key indicators of elder abuse, but these "lists" are based on studies of specific populations with varying definitions of types of abuse. Also, as research on elder abuse has grown, recent studies raise questions about factors that were identified as causes in earlier studies. For example, caregiver stress has been cited since the 1970s as an overarching cause of elder abuse, but elder abuse scholars currently emphasize that this narrow focus does not address societal conditions that have essential roles as causes of elder abuse, as discussed in Chapter 1. Another example is that elder abuse scholars are questioning gender stereotypes, emphasizing that men can frequently be victims and women can be perpetrators (Kosberg, 2014). The concluding message of a keynote presentation at the 7th World Conference of the International Network for the Prevention of Elder Abuse was that "attention should be directed not to gender, but to those conditions in different countries and cultures leading to abuse of both older men and women, including (but not limited to) economic problems, few alternatives to family care of the elderly, violence, changing characteristics of the family, ageism, and sexism" (Kosberg, 2014, p. 207).

Another consideration related to avoiding stereotypes about risks is that some studies identify increased prevalence of specific risks within certain groups, but these risks also occur—although with a lower frequency or to a lesser degree—in the general population of older adults. Risk factors may also be associated with certain groups in unique ways. For example, social isolation can be caused by stigma or prejudices associated with race, ethnicity, religion, sexual orientation, immigrant status, or other inherent characteristics. Language barriers or geographic location (e.g., rural) can also be sources of social isolation. For example, Vietnamese elders reported that daughters-in-law did not want them to learn English or use transportation so they could be confined at home to care for children and do household chores (Le, 1997).

Intergenerational Issues Related to Caregiving

Intergenerational issues related to caregiving are relevant to elder abuse in many ways. Major societal trends in the United States that affect the availability of family caregivers for older adults include increased life expectancy, increased employment of women, long-distance separation of older adults and younger family members, and increasing diversity of family constellations. These trends affect many White Americans, and a parallel trend affects American Indians (also referred to as Native Americans) who are experiencing not only the loss of caregiving support but also the loss of cultural connectivity when younger generations move to urban areas for financial and social reasons. Another cultural consideration is that intergenerational differences develop with immigrant older adults and their children who have grown up in the United States and become acculturated to new values that minimize filial responsibilities. For example, Asian older adults who gained entry as parents of U.S. citizens may live with children and grandchildren who have rapidly acculturated to mainstream values, creating intergenerational conflicts between expectations of the parents and attitudes of younger family members (Lee et al., 2014).

> Elder abuse is, first, alienating us because we are old. Kids tell us, "You mom and dad can't speak English so don't speak anything. Keep your mouths shut." It hurts a lot. It results in complete alienation. (Lee et al., 2014, p. 7)

Considerations Related to Immigrants and Language Barriers

Older adults who are immigrants may experience conditions that affect the risk for elder abuse, for example, because of social isolation. Language barriers, fear of deportation, and fear of involvement of public authorities may increase the risk for elder abuse being purposefully hidden by both the victim and the perpetrator. Older adults who enter the United States under sponsorship agreements may be particularly vulnerable to abuse because they are fearful of being deported if they do not cooperate with the family member who sponsored them. In addition, lack of linguistically appropriate services and actual and perceived racism and prejudice create barriers to services. The National Center on Elder Abuse provides educational materials on elder abuse in Spanish, Asian languages, and other languages, as illustrated in Figure 5.1.

Linguistic competence, which refers to health care services that are responsive to and respectful of a person's language abilities, is one small

FIGURE 5.1   Example of educational material on elder abuse in Spanish.

SEÑALES DE ALERTA DE MALTRATO

Alguien que usted conoce - una persona mayor o adulta con una discapacidad - ¿muestra alguna señal de alerta por maltrato?

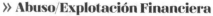

» Negligencia

- Falta de higiene básica, alimentos adecuados o ropa limpia y apropiada
- Falta de ayuda médica (gafas, andadera, dientes, ayuda auditiva, medicinas)
- Persona con demencia sin supervisión
- Persona confinada a la cama la dejan sin atención
- Casa desordenada, sucia, en mal estado o que tiene peligros de incendio y de seguridad
- Casa sin servicios adecuados (estufa, refrigerador, calefacción, ventilación, plomería y electricidad que funcionen)
- Llagas por presión de cama (úlceras de decúbito)

» Abuso/Explotación Financiera

- Falta de amenidades que la víctima pueda comprar
- Anciano/adulto vulnerable que "voluntariamente" da inusualmente reembolsos/regalos financieros excesivos para los cuidados necesarios y el compañerismo
- La persona que cuida de la persona anciana tiene control del dinero pero está fallando en proporcionar para lo necesario de la persona anciana
- Anciano/adulto vulnerable ha firmado transferencia de su propiedad (Carta-Poder, nuevo testamento, etc.) pero no puede comprender la transacción ni la que significa

» Abuso Psicológico/Emocional

- Cambios inexplicables o no característicos en comportamiento, tales como abandono de actividades normales, cambios bruscos de su estado de alerta u otros cambios
- El cuidador aísla a la persona anciana (no permite que alguien entre al hogar o hable con la persona anciana)
- El cuidador es verbalmente agresivo o humillante, controlador, excesivamente inquieto o desinteresado sobre gastar el dinero

» Abuso Físico/Sexual

- Fracturas, moretones, verdugones, cortaduras, llagas o quemaduras sin explicación adecuada
- Enfermedades trasmitidas sexualmente sin explicación

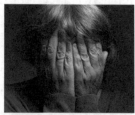

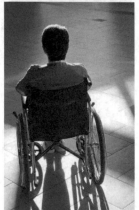

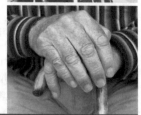

Si usted o alguien que usted conoce está en una situación que le amenace la vida o en peligro inmediato, llame al **911** o a la policía o alguacil local.

(continued)

part of cultural competence. This is particularly important in actual or suspected elder abuse situations involving older adults who rely on family members for communicating on their behalf. In these situations, it is imperative to use professional interpreter resources because it is difficult to know what the role of a family member or caregiver is in perpetrating, supporting, or ignoring abuse of the older adult. Since 2001, the

FIGURE 5.1   Example of educational material on elder abuse in Spanish. *(continued)*

¿QUÉ ES MALTRATO DE ANCIANOS?

En general, el abuso de ancianos se refiere a actos intencionales o desidiosos por parte del cuidador o la persona "de confianza" que lleva a o podría llevar a daño de un anciano vulnerable. *En muchos estados, los jóvenes adultos con discapacidades pueden calificar para el mismo servicio y protecciones.* **El maltrato físico; la desatención; el abuso emocional o psicológico; el abuso financiero y la explotación; el abuso sexual; y el abandono** se consideran formas de maltrato de ancianos. En muchos estados, el **descuido de sí mismo** es también considerado como maltrato.

¿QUIENES ESTÁN EN RIESGO?

El maltrato de ancianos puede suceder *en cualquier parte* - en el hogar, en un sanatorio o cualquier otro instituto. Afecta a las personas mayores de todos los grupos socioeconómicos, culturales y razas.

Basándose en información disponible, las mujeres y ancianos "más viejos" son los más propensos a ser victimizados. La demencia es un factor importante de riesgo. Los problemas de salud mental y abusos de sustancia - tanto de abusadores como de víctimas - son factores de riesgo. El aislamiento también puede contribuir al riesgo.

¿QUÉ DEBO HACER SI SOSPECHO DE ABUSO?

Reporte sus inquietudes.

La mayoría de los casos de maltrato de ancianos pasan sin ser detectados. No suponga que alguien ha reportado ya una situación sospechosa. La agencia que recibe el reporte le preguntará qué fue lo que usted observó, quiénes estaban involucrados y con quién se pueden comunicar para saber más.

Usted no tiene que probar que está sucediendo un abuso; es cuestión de los profesionales investigar las sospechas.

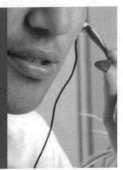

》 **Para reportar sospecha de abuso en la comunidad**, entre en contacto con su agencia local de Servicios de Protección de Adultos. Para los números donde reportar, visite **www.apsnetwork.org**, visite la página web de **NCEA** en **www.ncea.aoa.gov** o llame a *Eldercare Locator* al **1-800-677-1116 (eldercare.gov)**.

》 **Para reportar sospecha de abuso en un asilo de ancianos o centro de cuidados a largo plazo**, contacte a su Defensor local de Pueblo de Cuidados a Largo Plazo. Para los números donde reportar, visite **www.ltcombudsman.org**, visite la página web de NCEA al **www.ncea.aoa.gov** o llame al *Eldercare Locator* al **1-800-677-1116 (eldercare.gov)**.

El **Centro Nacional para Abuso de Ancianos (NCEA)** dirigido por la Administración de Envejecimiento de los EEUU, ayuda a las comunidades, las agencias y las organizaciones garantizar que los ancianos y los adultos con discapacidades puedan vivir con dignidad y sin abuso, desatención y explotación. NCEA es el lugar para acudir en busca de **educación, investigación y prácticas prometedoras para detener el abuso**.

Keck School of Medicine of USC

¡Visítenos en línea para ver más recursos! **www.ncea.aoa.gov**
Encuéntrenos en Facebook y Twitter.

Este documento fue completado para el Centro Nacional para Abuso de Ancianos y está apoyado en parte por un subsidio (No. 90AB0002/01 UCI Center of Excellence) de la Administración sobre Envejecimiento del Departamento de Salud y Servicios Humanos (DHHS) de los EEUU. A los concesionarios que llevan a cabo los proyectos bajo el patrocinio del gobierno se les anima a expresar libremente sus hallazgos y conclusiones. De manera que, los puntos de vista u opiniones no representan necesariamente la política oficial de la Administración sobre Envejecimiento o DHHS.

El Centro de Excelencia está agradecido a sus generosos partidarios: la fundación Archstone Foundation, el Instituto Nacional de Justicia, el Instituto Nacional sobre Envejecimiento, la fundación UniHealth Foundation y los donadores individuales.

Source: National Center on Elder Abuse.

federal government has required all health care institutions that receive federal funds (including all Medicare and Medicaid nursing homes) to provide access to 24-hour, no-cost language assistance services for individuals who have limited English-language abilities.

Whenever nurses suspect elder abuse, they need to advocate for the use of language assistance services, even though it may be more

A 75-year-old woman was forced to work in a restaurant from four in the morning till four in the afternoon and then go home and cook for her family and look after the children . . . on a sponsorship. Older immigrants have been threatened with all kinds of things. (Walsh, Olson, Ploeg, Lohfeld, & Macmillan, 2011, p. 31)

An 82-year-old East European lady with limited English had been in a marriage for over 30 years. . . . There was constant psychological abuse and he basically kept her as a personal slave. . . . She had absolutely no money. . . . Several times she ended up in the hospital because of the beatings. She didn't know where to turn for help. (Walsh, Olson, Ploeg, Lohfeld, & Macmillan, 2011, p. 33)

convenient to accept the interpretations provided by families or others involved with the situation. Hospitals and medical centers usually post information for language assistance services in public places, but it may be more difficult to find appropriate services in other settings. When elder abuse is suspected in community settings, nurses can call local adult protective service organizations or culturally specific organizations to inquire about bilingual staff or resources. When elder abuse is suspected in long-term care settings, the local Long-Term Care Ombudsman program may have bilingual staff or be able to provide information about interpreters if the facility does not do so. In these situations, the nursing home ombudsman should be contacted as a third party because the resources provided by the long-term care facility may not be objective. In all health care settings, nurses can inquire about access to language assistance services that are mandated by federal regulations.

RELEVANCE FOR NURSES

Current realities and trends related to diversity in the United States point to the necessity of all health care professionals incorporating cultural competence in caring for clients and patients. Nurses can develop cultural competence related to dimensions of elder abuse by considering questions such as the ones described in Box 5.1. Nurses cannot answer all of these questions in any patient-care situation, but they can mentally integrate these types of questions in their assessments of older adults and family caregivers. These questions also serve as a guide to developing an awareness of the many ways in which cultural dimensions may be influencing perceptions of and risks for elder abuse.

BOX 5.1 Cultural Considerations Pertinent to Dimensions of Elder Abuse

Considerations related to nursing assessment and interventions

- How am I influenced by any of the following: ageism, my own cultural background, my personal experiences, and my attitudes about caregiving?
- How do my views and experiences affect my perceptions of abuse and violence?
- How might lack of knowledge about culturally diverse groups influence my nursing care of older adults and their caregivers?
- Am I careful about avoiding stereotypes and generalizations related to older adults, caregivers, and elder abuse?
- What interventions can I use to address conditions such as low health literacy and language barriers?
- How do cultural factors affect the use of resources that I might suggest?

Roles of older adults within the family and community

- How have traditional cultural values influenced perceptions of roles of older adults, and do these differ across generations?
- What current factors influence roles of older adults within the family?

Expectations related to interpersonal relationships

- What conduct is considered abusive in the family, by the community, and in the country of the person's origin?
- How do culturally based views of gender roles influence the perception of spousal and interfamilial relationships between men and women?
- How do one's past and present experiences—on personal, familial, environmental, and societal levels—influence one's perceptions of violence in general and in interpersonal relationships specifically?

Perceptions of autonomy and independence versus safety and dependency

- Does ageism or other factors influence perceptions of an older adult's right to choose to live in situations involving risks to safety?
- Do family members differ in their perceptions of the older adult's right to make decisions about his or her care?

(continued)

BOX 5.1 Cultural Considerations Pertinent to Dimensions of Elder Abuse *(continued)*

Expectations about family caregiving
- How are decisions made about the provision of care for older adults who need assistance?
- Who within the family is expected to care for frail and dependent older members and what happens if they fail to do so?
- Is it acceptable to employ paid caregivers?
- Do family members differ in their perceptions of caregiving responsibilities, especially across generations?
- How might cultural perspectives influence the roles of family related to expectations for caregiving?
- Are older grandparents expected to care for grandchildren and great-grandchildren?

Decisions about family resources
- How might cultural perspectives influence family expectations related to financial support across generations?
- Who makes decisions about how family resources are expended?
- Who, within the family, is expected to provide financial support for older members?
- Does the family consider it appropriate to use the older member's resources for the benefit of other family members?

Attitudes about using nonfamily resources
- How do religious beliefs, past experiences, and attitudes affect decisions about accepting services from outsiders?
- What are the acceptable sources of help from outsiders (e.g., extended family, religious leaders, respected members of the community, healers within their community)?

Considerations related to sources of information
- What are the trusted sources of information in the community?
- How is the older adult's ability to obtain reliable information affected by low literacy or limited language?

(continued)

BOX 5.1   Cultural Considerations Pertinent to Dimensions of Elder Abuse (*continued*)

Considerations related to immigrant older adults or those with communication barriers

- When did the older and younger generations of the family come to the United States (e.g., together or at different times, which generation came first)?

- What were the circumstances of immigration for the different members of the family?

- Were there sponsorship agreements between the older and younger family members, and, if so, what were the expectations related to financial or caregiving support?

- What is the legal status of the older adults and other members of the family?

- Do communication barriers influence the care that is provided or limit the caregiving resources?

Considerations related to nursing assessment of physical abuse

- How does skin color affect assessment of bruises, pressure sores, and other skin changes?

CULTURAL DIVERSITY IN THE UNITED STATES AND ITS RELEVANCE TO ELDER ABUSE

The federal government provides information about older adults in four ethnic and racial groups, with each group including multiple and diverse subgroups, as described in the following sections. Although the information about ethnic and racial groups is narrow and "generic," it provides a statistical profile of the population of older adults in the United States. In 2014, more than one of five older adults in the United States are members of the following racial or ethnic groups: 9% African Americans, 8% Hispanic, 4% Asian, and 0.5% American Indian. By 2060, the U.S. Census Bureau projects that 44% of older adults will belong to one of these four major ethnic or racial groups: 12% African Americans, 22% Hispanic, 9% Asian, and 1% American Indian (U.S. Census Bureau, Population Division, 2014).

In addition to ethnic and racial characteristics, diversity needs to be considered within many other contexts including the following: gender; sexual identity; socioeconomic status; educational level; health literacy; geographic setting (e.g., rural, urban, Indian Country); marital status; citizenship status in the United States; first-, second-, or third-generation immigration status; and experiences of trauma and violence in immediate and past communities and relationships.

Common Themes Related to Elder Abuse in Culturally Specific Groups

Several themes recur in the literature about elder abuse in specific groups, particularly with regard to obligations to provide care for older family members and place the needs of the family over those of the individual members (i.e., "familism"). For example, research on African Americans, Asians, Latino, and American Indian caregivers has found that a strong sense of family obligation is associated with caregiving, in contrast to White caregivers (Goins et al., 2010). A related theme cited in many studies is that "sending an elderly parent to a nursing home was considered abusive across all of the sampled racial and ethnic and age groups because of cultural beliefs in filial piety and family-based elder care" (Lee et al., 2014).

Many cultural groups hold a strong sense of family self-reliance and tradition of resolving conflicts within the family. This cultural value promotes feelings of shame and a need to maintain secrecy about mistreatment by family members. Themes related to disrespect for elders are also common and are often manifest in culturally specific ways. For example, Asian older adults report experiences of "silent treatment" as a form of mistreatment by families.

> Certain things happen to you, you take it to the grave with you, you don't tell anyone, you're too ashamed and all that. (Bowes, Ghizala, & Macintosh, 2012, p. 268)

> Our people really worry about what the community will think. They don't want their son's or daughter's or their whole family's honor to be tarnished in any way. People will just accept the abuse, they will remain silent. (Bowes et al., 2012, p. 268)

The next four sections describe cultural considerations related to major ethnic and racial groups in the United States. The purpose of these is not to emphasize differences, but to provide information that is relevant to identifying and addressing elder abuse in culturally diverse groups. As with all information in this chapter, it is imperative to avoid stereotypes and see through the perspective of each individual older adult who may be at risk for or a victim of elder abuse as well as that of caregivers who are at risk for becoming a perpetrator.

CULTURAL CONSIDERATIONS RELATED TO ELDER ABUSE AND AFRICAN AMERICANS

Overview of African American Older Adults

African Americans are mainly the descendants of more than 20 million Africans who were forcibly brought to the United States as slaves in the beginning of the 17th century. This unique history is associated with inherent effects that remain today, including racism, poverty, and significant disparities in socioeconomic conditions. The high rates of poverty may lead to greater financial strain for African American families and greater risk for experiencing financial abuse (as discussed in Chapter 15). African Americans also experience health disparities that are associated with poor health, increased levels of disability, and decreased life expectancy. In addition, the unique experiences of injustices and exploitation carried out within the medical system (e.g., the Tuskegee syphilis experiment) foster a distrust of public institutions, including health care providers, in African Americans. An implication for care of older adults is that fear of nursing home placement has been found to be particularly strong among African Americans because nursing facilities are associated with elder abuse (Enguidanos, DeLiema, Aguilar, Lambrinos, & Wilber, 2014).

One positive consequence of the historical context is that African Americans tend to have a strong support network within their community and a high rate of participation in religious activities. Heo and Koeske (2011) suggest that prior experiences with adversity and cultural traditions of family caregiving are factors that improve coping abilities of African American caregivers. African American older adults have the highest level of religious participation, with the most common affiliations being Baptist, Methodist, Pentecostal, and Catholic (Chatters, Nguyen, & Taylor, 2014).

Geographic considerations associated with increased risk for elder abuse are that African Americans who live in rural areas may be socially isolated and those who live in urban areas are often exposed to high crime and substandard housing. For example, an African American urban middle-class and working-class focus group described physically violent and criminal actions by strangers as a common type of elder mistreatment (Dakin & Pearlmutter, 2009).

Perspectives of African Americans on Older Adults and Elder Abuse

African Americans have a strong tradition of holding their elders in high esteem, a deep sense of family loyalty, a reliance on family members in times of need and crisis, and a strong sense of preserving family unity during any challenge (Horsford, Parra-Cardona, Post, & Schiamberg, 2011). African American households are often multigenerational and headed by a female. In recent decades, there have been an increasing number of African American "skipped-generation" households in which grandparents are responsible for care of grandchildren who are younger than 18 years. For example, in 2012, almost 47.6% of these African American grandparents were responsible for care of grandchildren (U.S. Census Bureau, 2012). In these situations, the adult children and grandchildren may become perpetrators of financial exploitation, psychological abuse, or any other type of domestic abuse.

Obligations to care for a family member take precedence over personal needs and African American older adults may want their children nearby even if they are being abused by them (Mouton, 2013). One study found that African Americans who cared for an older adult would not label themselves as "caregivers" and they acknowledged the need for education related to caring for older relatives (Enguidanos et al., 2014). African American older adults may be reluctant to report abuse because they do not want to harm their family's reputation in the community, or be seen as going against their kin (Mouton, 2013). These characteristics are a strength in many ways, but they also lead to the belief that elder abuse and neglect are inadmissible behaviors in the African American community (Horsford et al., 2011).

Because they don't see what they are doing as abuse; it might be pointed out to them that this might not be the best way to resolve a situation. They have maternity classes for teenage mothers because they don't know how to take care of a baby, and we don't know how to take care of an elderly. (Enguidanos et al., 2014, p. 11)

Implications for Nurses

Long-lasting effects of oppression, racism, discrimination, exploitation, and exclusion continue to affect the lives of African Americans in many ways. An implication for nurses is that African Americans may distrust health care providers and organizations and this may interfere with acceptability of services to prevent or address elder abuse. A question such as "Whom can you turn to when you need help?" may

help identify resources that are acceptable for addressing situations that are
actually or potentially abusive. It is
important to ask older adults about
any network of "kinfolk" who can be
involved with providing care. Ministers
and other people associated with religious organizations (e.g., Faith Community Nurses) have important roles as
support resources. Additional sources
of support may be found through local
senior centers and caregiver support

> If you understand where I'm
> coming from culturally and what
> is happening to me, where I am
> in my aging process. If you got
> those two pieces together, then
> you'd have the foundation for a
> beginning relationship. (71-year-
> old African American woman;
> Hansen, Hodgson, & Gitlin,
> 2015, p. 7)

groups. It may be appropriate to avoid referring to family as "caregivers" but simply refer to them as "family" or "kin."

Resources for Information About Elder Abuse and African American Older Adults

National Center on Elder Abuse, www.ncea.aoa.gov

- Publishes research brief on "Elder Abuse in the African
  American Community"

Alzheimer's Association, www.alz.org

- Provides educational materials specific for African American
  caregivers

CULTURAL CONSIDERATIONS RELATED TO LATINO OLDER ADULTS

Overview of Latino American Older Adults

The federal government category of *Latino Americans* (also called *Hispanic Americans)* includes many heterogeneous groups that have immigrated to the United States from Mexico (64.0%), Puerto Rico (9.4%), El
Salvador (3.8%), Cuba (3.7%), the Dominican Republic (3.1%), Guate-
mala (2.3%), and many other countries (less than 2% each; U.S. Census
Bureau News, 2014). Although these groups share some common characteristics, they represent culturally diverse subgroups that are combined for reasons such as census and research. Older Latino Americans
are likely to be poor, have less than a high school level of education,

and speak Spanish in their homes. They also tend to hold strong religious beliefs, including finding meaning in suffering and a tendency to suffer in silence as a coping strategy (Chatters et al., 2014). Much of the research on Latino older adults has been done on Mexican Americans.

Perspectives of Latino Americans on Older Adults and Elder Abuse

Latinos have high regard (*respecto*) for people by virtue of their age, service, or experience, and this carries over to a strong sense of respect for older adults. They also have a strong sense of family (*familia*), which emphasizes the needs of family over the needs of the individual. This cultural value can hinder the reporting of elder abuse as well as the use of support services by Latino immigrants who depend on their families for care (DeLiema, Gassoumis, Homeier, & Wilber, 2012). Similarly, having a family member admitted to a nursing home goes against cultural norms related to family unity, respect for elders, and family obligations to care for aging parents.

The National Center on Elder Abuse (2014) identifies the following cultural factors that are related to increased risk for and lack of reporting elder abuse in Latino Americans:

- Female gender role expectations of *marianismo* (i.e., feminine passivity and moral strength) mandating women to tolerate abuse and accept violent partnerships as commonplace

- Male gender role expectation of *machismo* (i.e., male superiority and strong sense of masculine pride), which prevents a male elder from revealing mistreatment because of the associated loss of respect and status

- *Verguenzaza*, shame and embarrassment, which promotes tolerance of family violence and interferes with reporting and acceptance of services

- Intergenerational economic dependency and cultural beliefs about sharing family money and resources may influence perceptions of financial abuse

- Limited English, lack of citizenship, fear of deportation, and general mistrust of government interferes with reporting and acceptance of services

Testimony at the U.S. Senate Special Committee on Aging emphasized that Latino elder abuse victims often face intersecting issues that compound the problem, such as racism, economic barriers, language barriers, acculturation issues, social isolation, anti-immigrant sentiment, and challenges dealing with the criminal justice system (Lee, Kaplan, & Perez-Stable, 2014).

Implications for Nurses

Latino American older adults may distrust health care services and be reluctant to accept services because they want to avoid exposure to the legal or immigration system. Even those who are in the United States legally may fear the exposure of other relatives who may not be legal immigrants, especially if they live in a state that fosters anti-immigration laws or policies. Thus, it is important to establish trust by communicating a nonjudgmental attitude. Culturally appropriate communication with older Hispanic Americans typically involves showing respect by addressing the older adult by using a salutation that includes his or her last name and beginning a conversation through an exchange of pleasantries or social topics. Also, it is important to avoid any implication that family caregivers are not providing good care.

Perspectives of older Latino Americans with regard to using outside services may differ significantly from those of younger family members. When discussing plans for care, focus on the specific needs of the older adult and identify resources that are available to address these needs. Asking about religious or spiritual supports may help identify resources for acceptable services. For example, a question such as "Do you identify with any religious group in your community?" may open the door for additional questions such as "Does that church have any services that might be helpful to you and your family when you are home from the hospital?" In addition, it may be helpful to acknowledge an older adult's sadness about the inability of family to provide the required care and assure the older adult that the use of outside services or a long-term care facility is not necessarily an indicator of a family member's lack of love and respect.

> Foreign-born Latino elders referred to the United States as "a country of opportunities for younger people, but not a place to grow old, because old people are not respected and valued." (Beyene, Becker, & Mayen, 2002, p. 166)

Resources for Information on Elder Abuse and Latino Americans

Casa de Esperanza, www.casadeesperanza.org

■ Federally funded National Culturally Specific Special Issue Resource Center that focuses on working within Latino communities for prevention and intervention efforts to address domestic violence

- Provides support, education, and assistance through local domestic violence hotlines
- Addresses rights of immigrants who are victims of domestic violence through local organizations

National Center on Elder Abuse, www.ncea.aoa.gov

- Provides Spanish-language resources for teaching patients and families about elder abuse

National Hispanic Council on Aging (NHCOA), www.nhcoa.org

- Provides services through local Hispanic Aging Network centers throughout the United States

CULTURAL CONSIDERATIONS RELATED TO ELDER ABUSE AND ASIAN AMERICANS

Overview of Asian American Older Adults

Asian Americans (also called *Asians* and *Pacific Islanders*) is the term applied by the U.S. Census Bureau in reference to people who come from China, the Philippines, India, Vietnam, Korea, Japan, and other countries. The category is extremely heterogeneous and includes people from nearly 50 countries and ethnic groups who speak more than 100 languages and dialects (Social Security Administration, 2013). Asian Americans are very diverse with regard to reasons for migrating to the United States, ranging from those who came as laborers during the 1700s (Filipinos), 1800s (Chinese and Japanese), or 1900s (Koreans and Asian Indians) to those who came after 1970 seeking political refuge (Vietnamese). Despite this long history of immigration, significant gaps occurred when Chinese and Koreans were excluded from immigration to the United States beginning in the 1940s. Currently, more than two thirds of Asian Americans are foreign-born and the majority entered the United States during or after the 1990s.

The current group of Chinese and Korean older adults in the United States is characterized by low income levels, less than a high school education, social isolation within their ethnic communities, and low levels of acculturation and English-language skills (Lee, Moon, & Gomez, 2014). Some of these immigrants are older parents who have been brought to the United States by younger Asian American adults who have come for education and employment. Overall, more than two thirds of Asian American older adults do not speak English well and one half of Korean, Chinese, and Vietnamese older adults live in a household where English is not spoken (U.S. Census Bureau, 2012).

Perspectives of Asian Americans on Older Adults and Elder Abuse

Korean and Chinese immigrants who participated in a focus group identified the following interrelated dimensions of sociocultural values and beliefs that are integral to understanding the context of elder abuse: collectivism and family harmony, filial piety, gender roles and male dominance, spiritual and religious beliefs, and immigration and acculturation (Lee, Moon, et al., 2014). Asian communities have traditionally placed great value on the veneration of all elders, who hold tremendous authority and power in all spheres of family matters and important decision making. Despite this deep-rooted cultural tradition of respect for the elderly, recent research indicates that elder abuse is a pervasive health issue for Chinese American older adults (Dong, Chang, Wong, & Simon, 2013). Filial piety is a core philosophy of the teachings of Confucius, which prescribes adult children's obligatory roles and responsibilities of caregiving to aging parents. In return, parents are expected to contribute to the harmony of family and society with their guidance and wisdom. Thus, many Asian older adults expect to live with adult children, particularly the oldest son and his wife. If this does not occur, older adults may define this as abandonment, psychological abuse, or simply as elder abuse. This also has implications for definitions of financial exploitation because Asian families may be expected to provide care in return for transferring assets.

A related theme is that admitting to neglect and abuse means acknowledging one's weak capacity in self-protection and also admitting to others that family members are not fulfilling filial obligation of respecting elders (Lai, 2011). Thus, these behaviors are viewed as shameful and have a negative reflection on the older adults because of the culturally based feelings of being interconnected to others through mutually understood commitments (Dong, Chang, Wong, & Simon, 2012). This theme is magnified by the cultural value of resolving issues within the family rather than allowing outsiders to even know about problems. Research suggests that this sense of shame and cultural stigma about elder abuse may overshadow motivations to seek interventions and lead to feelings of helplessness, depression, and even suicidal ideation and behaviors (Chang & Dong, 2014).

Disrespect is viewed within the context of family relationships and encompasses a broad array of behaviors that violate basic Asian cultural values. Elder abuse scholars cite disrespect as the most common culturally specific form of elder abuse and as a form that is invisible under categories of elder abuse derived from a Western cultural perspective (Lai, 2011). For example, insufficient attention from daughters-in-law or direct expressions of disagreement with mothers-in-law are commonly cited as forms of elder abuse (Yan, 2014). Chinese and Korean Americans have identified psychological abuse (e.g., being disrespected and ignored) as the worst forms of elder abuse that they could experience (Lee, Moon, et al., 2014; Yan, 2014). Box 5.2 provides examples of elder mistreatment described by Korean and Chinese immigrants in the greater San Francisco metropolitan area.

> There is a saying in Chinese community that says if bad things happen in family you don't go outside and spread it. . . . So the only thing [an abused older woman] can do is try to be patient and try to forgive, and hopefully that will reduce the tensions between the family members. (Walsh et al., 2011, p. 29)

Implications for Nurses

Asian older adults are more likely to respond to questions about their experiences of elder abuse if there are no negative ramifications for family or perpetrator. Thus, it is imperative to be sensitive to perceptions of shame and avoid implications that family is not providing care. Rather than using the term *abuse*, frame questions in the context of feeling "respected." For example, a question such as "Do you ever feel disrespected?" may elicit information about the older adult's perception of elder abuse, which may differ from definitions that are based on Western perspectives. It is also important to recognize that perceptions of Asian immigrants may differ significantly from those of younger family members, particularly those who came to the United States before their parents immigrated. For example, Asian older adults may consider it disrespectful if their adult children treat them as equals, and this has important implications for decision making related to care plans.

Although common themes can be identified in cultural dimensions of elder abuse among Asian Americans, these can vary significantly,

BOX 5.2 Korean and Chinese Immigrants Describe Their Perceptions of Elder Mistreatment

Filial Piety and Respect

- "The elders who came from Mainland China believed in 'Raising a child for old age.' Chinese culture is different from Western culture where most children leave their parents at age 18. Since the parents push their children out early, they should not expect their children to come back to take care of elders. . . . Chinese parents expect their children to love and take care of them as they take care of their children before."

- "The Westerners talk to their parents equally, saying 'You.' If you say that to your Korean parents, it is a disaster."

Verbal and Psychological Abuse

- "There is a husband. Whenever he gets drunk, he says to his wife, 'Get out of this house right now, so I can live with a new, young wife. You don't cook well, you cannot do anything good. You are ignorant and know nothing.' The wife does everything from house chores, obsessively cleaning, and cooking. Although he does not beat her up physically, he swears and uses bad languages that are extremely hurtful."

Male Dominance

- "It is a cultural difference. . . . We Korean immigrants maintain the same values we had when we entered the U.S., like the values of male dominance—a husband controls a wife's life."

Abandonment and Neglect

- "The daughter-in-law needs to go to work and once conflicts came up, she left the mother-in-law in Oakland alone. The elderly woman was not able to speak English. Luckily, she knew one word, 'Chinese,' so the policeman called many places where Chinese people live, and finally found that her son lived in San Francisco."

- "I saw a daughter who lives with her mother. When the son-in-law goes to work, he leaves his mother-in-law at Portsmouth Square every day, even on a rainy day. She wanders around and there is nothing to eat. . . . It is bad she pushes her mother out."

(continued)

BOX 5.2 Korean and Chinese Immigrants Describe Their Perceptions of Elder Mistreatment *(continued)*

Perspectives on Disclosure and Seeking Help

- "One thing is very purely cultural. There are Asian sayings that you keep your problems within your own family. Chinese and Korean thinking are different from Western thinking. They don't want to talk about it, they don't want to expose it, and the only time when elder abuse surfaces is when it reaches a crisis."

- "There must be some way to seek help, but we do not like to get help. We want to take all responsibility on our own. Endurance with patients, you know, we grew up with Confucianism. So we just put up with it. We suffer abuse, but it is like spitting in my face. It's my own fault that I raised my children like that."

- "We control ourselves, keep things inside and be quiet. We all show high self-esteem in public, not showing abuse at all."

- "I know of a son who is a dentist and quite famous in the Korean community. But we find that he beats his parents up physically until they can't bear it anymore. But they do not want their children to be punished for his face and honor. If the White American parents get hurt from their children physically, they will call the police. For them, only individualism matters. But the Korean parent will say, 'Let's drop it, let's keep it a secret.'"

Sources: Lee, Moon, et al. (2014). Reproduced with permission of The Haworth Maltreatment & Trauma Press via Copyright Clearance Center. (Taylor & Francis Ltd, http://www.tandfonline.com).

particularly in families that have been in the United States for several generations. For example, a study found that later-generation Japanese caregivers could maintain a level of filial responsibility toward a parent who was in a long-term care facility by visiting daily and providing companionship (Miyawaki, 2015). Culturally based services for older adults, including all levels of long-term care facilities, are increasingly available in metropolitan areas where there are large populations of Chinese or Japanese Americans. Nurses can suggest that Asian older adults and their families explore these resources to address their needs and reduce the risk for elder abuse.

Resources for Information Related to Elder Abuse and Asian Americans

National Center on Elder Abuse, www.ncea.aoa.gov

- Publishes research brief on "Mistreatment of Asian Pacific Islander (API) Elders," with details about cultural considerations for assessment of API elder mistreatment
- Provides culturally specific resources for teaching patients and families about elder abuse in Korean, Chinese, Vietnamese, and Tagalog (Filipino) languages

National Asian Pacific Center on Aging, www.napca.org

- Provides a only toll-free Asian-language helpline to provide language assistance for Chinese, Korean, and Vietnamese older adults

CULTURAL CONSIDERATIONS RELATED TO ELDER ABUSE AND AMERICAN INDIANS

Overview of American Indian Older Adults

The 2010 U.S. Census defines *American Indians and Alaska Natives* as people who descended from any of the original people of North, South, or Central America, and who maintain their tribal affiliation or community attachment. The term *Indian Country* is relevant to elder abuse because it defines boundaries for legal and programmatic considerations. As defined in federal law, Indian Country includes all lands within Indian reservations, all dependent Indian communities within the borders of the United States, and all Indian allotments. In July 2015, there were 567 federally recognized tribes, with each one having its own language, cultural traditions, and legal codes.

American Indian older adults have lived through a history that includes the experience of being forced to attend boarding schools, laws banning spiritual practices, and the societal belief that Indian culture was unacceptable (Smyer & Clark, 2011). Consequences of this unique history that remain today—and are associated with increased risk for elder abuse—include lower educational levels and significantly higher rates of the following: crime, poverty, substance abuse, multigenerational dependency, and major health disparities (e.g., disproportionately high rates of chronic conditions and physical disabilities). In addition, older American Indians experience intergenerational anger and grief associated with the loss of cultural and spiritual knowledge that elders have traditionally passed on to younger generations.

Older American Indians are likely to be poor, live in rural areas, have less than a high school level of education, and speak an indigenous language rather than English. They are the only ethnic group with greater representation in rural than in urban areas, with high concentrations in the Great Plains of the West, Alaska, and Hawaii (National Rural Health Association, 2013). American Indians are affected by many health disparities, particularly among those who reside in rural areas. Risk factors associated with elder abuse include social isolation, lack of support resources, high rates of chronic illness and functional limitations, high rates of substance abuse, and interdependency among generations combined with limited resources.

American Indians in rural areas, including reservations, rarely have access to community-based services, despite their increased need due to higher rates of disability and chronic conditions. In many situations, relatives care for elderly American Indians in their homes at great physical and emotional cost to the elder and the family members (Smyer & Clark, 2011). Reasons that American Indians are admitted to tribally owned nursing homes include any or all of the following: physical abuse of older adults by alcohol-abusing family members, alcohol abuse by the older adults themselves, and difficulty of family members providing care for older adults with cognitive impairment and/or psychiatric disorders (Choi, 2014). American Indians who live on reservations and require long-term care may need to relocate to an urban-area nursing home, where they are socially isolated from their families and communities and the care is not culturally or linguistically appropriate.

Unique Legal Aspects of Elder Abuse in Indian Country

American Indians who live in areas designated as Indian Country have unique legal issues related to elder abuse because each Indian tribe or nation maintains tribal sovereignty. Tribes began enacting elder abuse codes during the 1980s, but even among those tribes who do have elder abuse codes, few have the services to report, investigate, and intervene in elder abuse situations. During the early 2000s, federal agencies and American Indian organizations began addressing elder abuse research and prevention in Indian Country. In 2011, the National Indigenous Elder Justice Initiative (NIEJI) was established to address the lack of culturally appropriate information on elder abuse and to support the development of elder abuse codes specific for their tribes. These efforts are ongoing; however, in 2015, fewer than 9% of the federally recognized tribes in the United States had an elder abuse code. A goal of the 2014 to 2017 cycle of federal funding is to provide elder abuse training modules that reflect American Indian cultural values.

Tribal codes are similar to adult protective services codes in some ways, for example, by creating "elderly protection teams" to respond to cases of elder abuse. In other ways, however, they reflect the unique cultural traditions of American Indians. For example, some codes state that "no person shall be deemed to be abused for the sole reason that they are being furnished traditional remedial treatment by spiritual means" (Jackson & Sappier, 2005, p. 11). In addition, tribal codes describe culturally specific approaches to domestic elder abuse, as in the following example involving a Navajo Peacemaker session mandated by the Family Court Judges:

> An adult son, who under the influence of alcohol, has battered his mother. The entire family is included in the session, including the son's girlfriend, parents, brother and sister-in-law. After much discussion and soul searching, the son promises not to hit his mother again and not to use alcohol. (Jackson & Sappier, 2005)

American Indian elders have cited traditional practices that are no longer effective for addressing elder abuse. For example, abusers were ostracized, reprimanded, or banished, but these sanctions are no longer used. The traditional practice of the chief leading a family council is viewed as not having "much impact since most traditional leaders are also involved in a dysfunctional family" (Jackson & Sappier, 2005, p. 43). Elder abuse in Indian Country is being addressed by developing tribal codes, coordinating efforts with local and state adult protective service agencies, and using resources of the NIEJI.

Perspectives of American Indians on Elder Abuse

Traditionally, the family is the central unit of American Indian communities; elders are held in high esteem, and most families want to care for their elders in ways that preserve and promote their dignity and honor cultural traditions. However, a recurring theme in discussions

Our elders, preserving our past in their memories, influencing our present when we dare to listen, aiming us toward our future, rooted in their wisdom, they deserve our respect, not our abuse. (Pueblo of Laguna Elderly Code, cited in Jackson & Sappier, 2005, p. 1)

of elder abuse and American Indians is that things are changing and American Indian families and communities are becoming increasingly dysfunctional. Although violence against other tribal members is viewed as a threat to internal spiritual harmony, victimization and abuse of elders is currently recognized as a clandestine but increasing problem in the American Indian community (Smyer & Clark, 2011). This theme was reflected in the testimony of the director of the NIEJI at the 2015 White House Conference on Aging:

> Elder abuse is not our culture. Historically we have honored and respected our elders for they carry our culture and teachings. However, things have changed. Every time I speak to a group I have a line of people to talk to afterward who tell me stories of those they know and care about who are being abused or neglected in some way. They ask me what they can do or how they can be helped. (Gray, 2015)

Box 5.3 delineates examples of elder abuse as described by American Indian Elders and Tribal Judges.

Implications for Nurses

Nurses who provide care for American Indian older adults need to build trust and use culturally appropriate communication skills, particularly when the nurse and client or patient have different ethnic or racial backgrounds. This process involves allocating time for listening, which may be the most important process in working with American Indians (Barnard, 2007). Because American Indians do not consider themselves "abused," it is preferable to use terms such as *disrespected* or *bothered* (Gray, 2015). Another consideration is that services related to reporting and investigation of suspected elder abuse may differ for American Indian older adults who live in Indian Country. Nurses can find up-to-date information about tribal codes and hotlines for elder abuse in Indian Country at the NIEJI, as listed in the next section.

Interventions to address elder abuse in American Indian communities are more effective when they focus on indirect—rather than direct—approaches involving family and tribal members. For example, the federally funded American Indians Caregiver Program

BOX 5.3 Examples of Elder Abuse Described by American Indian Elders and Tribal Judges

Physical Abuse

- Assault and battery on a grandpa because he would not give his grandson the keys to his truck
- Drug taking and alcohol abuse leads to yelling and sometimes hitting elders

Neglect

- Failing to provide services or resources essential to the elder's practice of his customs, traditions, or religion
- Restraining elders from exercising their grandparents' rights

Spiritual Abuse

- Not including elders as leaders in traditional ceremonies
- Not allowing elders to share traditional teachings through stories
- Denying access to a traditional healer

Emotional Abuse

- Family members treating them as if they did not matter anymore
- Not listening when elders speak
- Not recognizing when elders are not receiving love and care
- Community not listening to elder concerns
- Grown children and grandchildren moving in with an elder, drinking, fighting, taking their money, and chasing caregivers away from the home

Exploitation

- Unreasonable imposition on the elder's time resources, such as leaving children or other persons in the care of the elder for extended

(continued)

BOX 5.3 Examples of Elder Abuse Described by American Indian Elders and Tribal Judges *(continued)*

periods of time or under circumstances in which the elder cannot adequately provide care
- Family gambled away elder's only income
- A grandmother raised two girls who are now adults and drug abusers. They moved back in with her and she is supporting them

Sexual Abuse

- Grandma was raped by her nephew. She would not talk about it because she was ashamed because it was her own nephew

Adapted from Jackson and Sappier (2005).

uses "family group counseling," based on the assumption that if families are involved and provided with adequate information, they can develop appropriate plans to deal with their own problems. This model uses "talking circles" of 12 to 15 people who are chosen by the elder and typically include friends, family, spiritual leaders, and one service provider. Nurses can explore the availability of these culturally specific interventions through the resources listed in the next section.

Resources for Information Related to Elder Abuse and American Indians

National Resource Center on Native American Aging, www.nrcnaa.org

■   Provides "Native Service Locator" information with details about and contacts for a wide range of tribal services for older adults

National Indigenous Elder Justice Initiative, www.nieji.org

■   Provides up-to-date information about tribal codes pertinent to elder abuse

■   Provides links to Internet resources related to elder abuse

Office for American Indian, Alaskan Native, and Native Hawaiian Programs, www.olderindians.aoa.gov

- Provides information about federally funded programs related to elder abuse (e.g., financial fraud in Indian Country)

KEY POINTS: WHAT NURSES NEED TO KNOW AND CAN DO

- Cultural factors influence all aspects of definitions, perceptions, and interventions related to situations of actual or potential elder abuse.
- Although evidence-based information about cultural dimensions of elder abuse is limited, it is important to learn about characteristics associated with minority and ethnic groups, while also avoiding stereotypes.
- It is imperative to use language assistance services for objective interpretation in all situations of actual or potential elder abuse.
- Think about questions delineated in Box 5.1 to develop cultural competence related to caring for older adults.
- Use resources described in this chapter to find information pertinent to culturally diverse groups of older adults.
- Explore local resources related to culturally diverse groups in the geographic area where you work.

REFERENCES

Barnard, A. (2007). Providing psychiatric-mental health care for Native Americans. *Journal of Psychosocial Nursing, 45*, 30–35.

Beyene, Y., Becker, G., & Mayen, N. (2002). Perception of aging and sense of well-being among Latino elderly. *Journal of Cross-Cultural Gerontology, 17*, 155–172.

Bowes, A., Avan, G., & Macintosh, S. B. (2012). Cultural diversity and the mistreatment of older people in Black and minority ethnic communities: Some implications for service provision. *Journal of Elder Abuse & Neglect, 24*, 251–274.

Chang, E., & Dong, X. (2014). Understanding elder abuse in the Chinese Community: The role of cultural, social, and community factors. *Elder abuse and its prevention: Workshop summary* (pp. 53–59). Washington, DC: National Academies Press.

Chatters, L. M., Nguyen, A. W., & Taylor, R. J. (2014). Religion and spirituality among older African Americans. In K. E. Whitfield & T. A. Baker (Eds.), *Handbook of minority aging* (pp. 47–64). New York, NY: Springer Publishing Company.

Choi, N. G. (2014). Racial/ethnic minority older adults in nursing homes: Need for culturally competent care. In K. E. Whitfield & T. A. Baker (Eds.), *Handbook of minority aging* (pp. 291–312). New York, NY: Springer Publishing Company.

Dakin, E., & Pearlmutter, S. (2009). Older women's perceptions of elder maltreatment and ethical dilemmas in adult protective services: A cross-cultural, exploratory study. *Journal of Elder Abuse & Neglect, 21,* 15–57.

DeLiema, M., Gassoumis, Z., Homeier, D., & Wilber, K. (2012). Determining prevalence and correlates of elder abuse using promotores: Low income immigrant Latinos report high rates of abuse and neglect. *Journal of the American Geriatrics Society, 60,* 1333–1339.

Dong, X., Chang, E.-S., Wong, E., & Simon, M. (2012). The perceptions, social dominants, and negative health outcomes associated with depressive symptoms among U.S. Chinese older adults. *Gerontologist, 52,* 650–663.

Dong, X., Chang, E.-S., Wong, E., & Simon, M. (2013). Perceived effectiveness of elder abuse interventions in psychological distress and the design of culturally adapted interventions: A qualitative study in the Chinese community in Chicago. *Journal of Aging Research, 2013.* doi:10.1155/2013/845245

Enguidanos, S., DeLiema, M., Aguilar, I., Lambrinos, J., & Wilber, K. (2014). Multicultural voices: Attitudes of older adults in the United States about elder mistreatment. *Ageing and Society, 34*(5), 877–903.

Goins, R. T., Spencer, S. M., McGuire, L. C., Goldberg, J., Wen, Y., & Henderson, J. A. (2010). Adult caregiving among American Indians: The role of cultural factors. *Gerontologist, 51,* 310–320.

Gray, J. (2015, May 6). *Testimony of Jacqueline S. Gray, PhD.* White House Conference on Aging, National Indigenous Elder Justice Initiative, Norman, OK.

Hansen, B. R., Hodgson, N. A., & Gitlin, L. N. (2015). It's a matter of trust: Older African Americans speak about their health care encounters. *Journal of Applied Gerontology.* doi:10.1177/0733464815570662

Heo, G. J., & Koeske, G. (2011). The role of religious coping and race in Alzheimer's disease caregiving. *Southern Gerontological Society, 32,* 582–604.

Horsford, S. R., Parra-Cardona, J., Post, L. A., & Schiamberg, L. (2011). Elder abuse and neglect in African American families: Informing practice based on ecological and cultural frameworks. *Journal of Elder Abuse & Neglect, 23,* 75–88.

Jackson, M. Y., & Sappier, T. (2005). *Elder abuse issues in Indian country.* Washington, DC: U.S. Department of Health and Human Services, Administration on Aging.

Jervis, L. L. (2014). Native elder mistreatment. In *Elder abuse and its prevention: Workshop summary* (pp. 75–79). Washington, DC: National Academies Press.

Kosberg, J. (2014). Rosalie Wolf Memorial Lecture: Reconsidering assumptions regarding men as elder abuse perpetrators and elder abuse victims. *Journal of Elder Abuse & Neglect, 26,* 207–222.

Lai, D. (2011). Abuse and neglect experienced by aging Chinese in Canada. *Journal of Elder Abuse & Neglect, 23,* 326–347.

Le, Q. K. (1997). Mistreatment of Vietnamese elderly by their families in the United States. *Journal of Elder Abuse & Neglect, 9,* 51–61.

Lee, Y.-S., Kaplan, C., & Perez-Stable, E. J. (2014). Elder mistreatment among Chinese and Korean immigrants: The roles of sociocultural contexts on perceptions and help-seeking behaviors. *Journal of Elder Abuse & Neglect, 26,* 244–269.

Lee, Y.-S., Moon, A., & Gomez, C. (2014). Elder mistreatment, culture, and help-seeking: A cross-cultural comparison of older Chinese and Korean immigrants. *Journal of Elder Abuse & Neglect, 26,* 244–269.

Miyawaki, C. E. (2015). Association of filial responsibility, ethnicity, and acculturation among Japanese American family caregivers of older adults. *Journal of Applied Gerontology, 1–24.* doi:10.1177/0733464815581484

Mouton, C. (2013, April). *Elder mistreatment in African Americans: Opportunities for prevention and treatment.* Presentation at Elder Abuse and Its Prevention: A Public Workshop of the Forum on Global Violence Prevention. Washington, DC.

National Center on Elder Abuse. (2014). Mistreatment of Latino Elders. Retrieved from www.ncea.aoa.gov

National Rural Health Association. (2013). *Elder health in rural America* [Policy brief]. Retrieved from www.RuralHealthWeb.org

Smyer, T., & Clark, M. C. (2011). A cultural paradox: Elder abuse in the Native American community. *Home Health Care Management & Practice, 23,* 201–206.

Social Security Administration. (2013). *Asian Americans and Pacific Islanders.* Retrieved from www.ssa.gov/aapi/index.htm

U.S. Census Bureau. (2012). *American Community Survey fact finder: Grandparents living with own grandchildren under 18 years (Black or African American).* Retrieved from www.census.gov

U.S. Census Bureau News. (2014). *Profile America. Facts for features: Hispanic heritage month, 2014* (Publication number CB14-FF.22). Washington, DC: U.S. Department of Commerce.

U.S. Census Bureau, Population Division. (2014). *Annual estimates of the resident population by sex, age, race alone or in combination, and Hispanic origin* for the United States and states: April 1, 2010 to July 1, 2013. In *A profile of older Americans: 2014*. Retrieved from www.aoa.gov

Walsh, C. A., Olson, J. L., Ploeg, J., Lohfeld, L., & Macmillan, H. L. (2011). Elder abuse and oppression: Voices of marginalized elders. *Journal of Elder Abuse & Neglect, 23*, 17–42.

Yan, E. (2014). Elder abuse in Asia: An overview. *Elder abuse and its prevention: Workshop summary* (pp. 105–122). Washington, DC: National Academies Press.

ROLES OF NURSES RELATED TO DETECTING AND REPORTING ELDER ABUSE

LAWS RELATED TO ELDER ABUSE AND ROLES OF NURSES AS REPORTERS

Although elder mistreatment has occurred in many ways throughout American history, elder abuse was not brought to public attention as a serious and widespread issue until the 1960s. The 1962 Public Welfare Amendments to the Social Security Act (SSA) is commonly cited as the initial milestone leading to the development of state-established adult protective services agencies (Teaster, Wangmo, & Anetzberger, 2010). Since then, scholars, legislators, public officials, and multiple professional groups—including nurses—have addressed elder abuse from many perspectives. Box 6.1 summarizes societal, professional, and legislative influences associated with the phases of progress related to elder abuse laws and programs.

Today, nurses in all settings need to not only be knowledgeable about reporting requirements related to suspected cases of elder abuse but also be able to find resources to help resolve these challenging situations. Throughout the United States, adult protective services programs are the fundamental resource for investigation and resolution of situations involving alleged abuse, neglect, or exploitation of vulnerable adults. This chapter presents information about legal responsibilities of nurses with regard to reporting suspected cases and describes resources that nurses can use to address older adults who are actual, potential, or suspected victims of elder abuse or neglect.

BOX 6.1   Phases of Progress Related to Elder Abuse and Adult Protective Services

1950s and 1960s: Discussion Phase

- Societal influences: increasing older population, geographic mobility of families
- Professional influences: scholarly discourse on protective services for mentally impaired older adults, recognition of need for multidisciplinary approach to problem resolution
- Federal legislation: 1962 SSA Public Welfare Amendments established protective services for persons with physical and/or mental limitations who were unable to manage their own affairs or who were neglected or exploited

1970s: Discovery Phase

- Societal influences: development of "rights" movements, expansion of the public service sector
- Professional influences: first federally supported research on elder abuse as a social problem; recognition of "battered old person syndrome" by Robert Butler, MD
- Federal legislation: 1974 SSA Title XX expanded funds for protective services for all adults age 18 and older without regard to income
- State laws: first adult protective services laws, with some including mandatory reporting and some including involuntary interventions (e.g., emergency orders, civil commitments)

1980s: Development Phase

- Societal influences: moral agendas and criminalization of unacceptable behaviors, movement away from entitlement programs
- Professional influences: pioneering research on elder abuse, establishment of organizations to support improved understanding of and response to elder abuse
- Publication of first books on elder abuse, including one co-authored by a nurse and social worker titled *Abuse and Maltreatment of the Elderly: Causes and Interventions* (Quinn & Tomita, 1986)

(continued)

BOX 6.1 Phases of Progress Related to Elder Abuse and Adult Protective Services *(continued)*

- Formation of the National Committee for the Prevention of Elder Abuse; publication of *Journal of Elder Abuse and Neglect*
- Federal legislation: 1987 Older Americans Act Amendments required states to provide services for preventing elder abuse, neglect, and exploitation; 1987 Nursing Home Reform Act required reporting of abuse of nursing home residents

1990s: Diversification Phase

- Societal influences: increasing awareness of domestic violence
- Professional influences: expanded conceptualization of elder abuse and the systems involved with addressing it, including public health departments
- Establishment of major organizations: National Center on Elder Abuse, International Network for the Prevention of Elder Abuse, and National Adult Protective Services Association
- Federal legislation: 1992 Vulnerable Elder Rights Protection Act authorized ombudsman programs to investigate allegations of elder abuse in long-term care settings; 1992 Family Violence Prevention and Services Act mandated the National Elder Abuse Incidence Study

2000–2015: Declaration Phase

- Societal influences: increasing use of social media, widespread acknowledgment of elder abuse and fraud, scams, and financial exploitation
- Professional influences: first nationally representative prevalence studies of elder abuse in the United States; emphasis on evidence-based practice, including research on "best practices" for preventing and treating elder abuse and neglect
- Development of the following: Administration on Aging's Year of Elder Abuse Prevention, Institute of Medicine's Elder Abuse Prevention Workshop, annual recognition of World Elder Abuse Awareness Day,

(continued)

BOX 6.1   Phases of Progress Related to Elder Abuse and
Adult Protective Services *(continued)*

identification of elder justice as one of four priority topics addressed
by the 2015 White House Conference on Aging

• Federal legislation: Protecting Seniors from Fraud Act (2000) provided
funds to educate seniors about scams and to develop strategies to
prevent financial crimes against seniors; Elder Justice Act (2010) established the Elder Justice Coordinating Council and provides limited
funding for state adult protective services and for research, training,
and new methods of dealing with elder abuse.

Adapted from Anetzberger (2004). Used with permission of author.

LAWS RELATED TO ELDER ABUSE

Since 1993, all 50 states and the District of Columbia have had laws
that do the following: (a) Define elder abuse and neglect; (b) apply to
suspected cases of elder abuse, neglect, or exploitation in domestic
settings; (c) describe a process for investigation; and (d) require a
response to the abuse and punishment of the abuse. These types of
laws are collectively referred to as *adult protective services laws* or *elder
abuse laws*. Initially, not all state laws included mandatory reporting
by health care professionals, but by 2015, New York was the only
exception to this. Elder abuse laws do not require reporters to *know*
whether abuse or neglect has occurred, but it does require them to
report it if they *suspect* its occurrence. The responsibility for problem
verification rests with the public agency charged with law implementation, not with the reporter or referral source.

All laws protect reporters from any form of retribution, as long as
the report is made in good faith. In addition, laws generally protect
the identity of the reporter, except as necessary among involved agencies. State laws also define penalties, such as fines or misdemeanor
charges, for mandatory reporters if they fail to report. In addition to
mandatory reporting of suspected cases by certain professions, all states
provide for voluntary reporting by anyone. Not all state laws include
provisions to punish the abuser; however, this issue is addressed in
separate criminal codes. Box 6.2 identifies variations in elder abuse

BOX 6.2 Variations in Elder Abuse Statutes Among 50 States and the District of Columbia

Types defined, either specifically or within general definition

- *Physical abuse, neglect, and financial or material exploitation* are identified in all statutes.
- *Emotional or psychological abuse* is identified in 44 statutes.
- *Self-neglect* is identified in 40 statutes.
- *Sexual abuse* is considered as a form of physical abuse and identified separately in 37 statutes.
- *Abandonment* is identified in 13 statutes.
- Some definitions of neglect include negligence, whereas others require a degree of willfulness.
- Some definitions of physical abuse distinguish between willful infliction and negligent failure to prevent the abuse.
- Some statutes require psychological abuse to be severe enough to require medical attention.
- A few states recognize unreasonable confinement; some include intimidation.
- Legally, abuse can occur under the general category of "violation of rights."

Groups defined as "protected" and residing in domestic settings

- Included population: vulnerable adult, older person, elderly adult, disabled person, endangered adult, at-risk adult, dependent adult in need of protective services
- Defined ages: 43 states include dependent adults, 18 and older, who lack decision-making capacity due to physical or mental illness, disability, or deficiency; other states define older adults at age 60 or 65

Types of state agencies designated to receive reports and investigate

- Aging-specific agency (e.g., Department of Aging, Department of Elder Affairs)
- Department or Commission of Human Services or Resources
- Department or Commission of Social Services
- Adult protective services
- Department of Public Health
- Law enforcement (e.g., police, sheriff, attorney general)

Adapted from Frolik and Kaplan (2014), and Jirik and Sanders (2014).

laws with regard to types, protected groups, and state agencies responsible for receiving reports and investigating. Appendix A lists state websites and phone numbers for reporting suspected cases. Helpful resources for information about reporting elder abuse are listed at the end of this chapter.

CONCERNS OF NURSES RELATED TO REPORTING

Although state and federal laws and regulations require nurses to report suspected cases of elder abuse, most nurses are uncomfortable with this responsibility for many reasons, including questions about confidentiality. The Health Insurance Portability and Accountability Act (HIPAA) of 1996 requires health care providers to obtain written permission from patients (or their designated representative in cases of inability or incompetence) before sharing information about the patient's condition. In situations of abuse, neglect, or domestic violence, the Department of Health and Human Services has clearly stated that health care professionals are permitted to share protected health information with appropriate authorities without the individual's permission (Campanelli, 2004). The agency that investigates the report ordinarily will not disclose the source of the report, except to other professionals involved and only as pertinent to the case. All agencies involved maintain confidentiality as much as possible.

Another concern is whether a nurse who makes a report should inform the older adult. Although federal regulations encourage reporters to inform the individual about the report, they also allow reporters to exercise professional judgment, particularly if the disclosure would increase the risk of harm or not be in the best interest of the alleged victim (Code of Federal Regulations, 2010).

In all states, responsibility for making the report rests with the individual nurse, who is responsible, also, for the consequences of failing to do so. Nurses have identified all the following conditions that contribute to the lack of reporting: more immediate and overriding priorities, alternative explanations for patient's conditions, lack of time, lack of knowledge or misperceptions about reporting responsibilities, difficulty obtaining privacy for talking alone with the older adult, inability to assess on an ongoing basis, negative experiences with adult protective services, and a tendency to report suspicions only to other professionals within their institutional settings (Schmeidel, Daly, Rosenbaum, Schmuch, & Jogerst, 2012).

All health care institutions accredited by the Joint Commission on Healthcare Organizations are required to implement policies and procedures for identifying, treating, and referring victims of abuse and to educate staff about domestic violence. It is imperative to recognize that domestic violence occurs across all age groups and affects men and women in any type of living arrangement. Box 6.3 addresses nurses' frequently asked questions about reporting. Chapter 7 discusses tools and guides used in detecting elder abuse, and Chapter 8 addresses ethical issues.

ADULT PROTECTIVE SERVICES

The National Adult Protective Services Association describes adult protective services as a social services program available nationwide to serve "seniors and adults with disabilities who are in need of assistance. Adult protective services workers frequently serve as first responders in cases of abuse, neglect or exploitation, working closely with a wide variety of allied professionals, such as physicians, nurses, paramedics, firefighters, and law enforcement officers" (National Adult Protective Services Organization, n.d.). Although the organization of and services provided by adult protective services agencies vary significantly, the common element is that they all "serve as first responders." Nurses and others who make reports do not have to *know* that elder abuse is occurring or has occurred, but they merely need to *suspect* it to initiate an adult protective services referral. In a nutshell, nurses are responsible for reporting and adult protective services agencies are responsible for investigating and substantiating what is reported. Figure 6.1 illustrates the general process used by adult protective services for addressing alleged elder abuse. Because the process is implemented at state and local levels, some aspects may vary, particularly with regard to eligibility criteria. For example, some states designate different reporting agencies depending on whether the situation occurs in a domestic setting or long-term care facility.

HELPFUL RESOURCES FOR INFORMATION ABOUT REPORTING

Many nonprofit and governmental agencies provide extensive information about elder abuse for professionals and nonprofessionals; these

BOX 6.3 Nurses' Frequently Asked Questions About Reporting

What if I think my report may place the elder in more danger?
Report actual or suspected cases for investigation, recognizing that it is
the responsibility of adult protective services to reduce the risk.

*How can I know that older adults at risk clearly understand the conse-
quences of their actions?*
These situations require a comprehensive evaluation of the person's
decision-making abilities. If this cannot be done while the person is
receiving care from you, it will be done by adult protective services
after a report is made.

*What do I do when I have concerns about the older adult following
discharge from my health care setting?*
When in doubt, you can consult with adult protective services about an
older adult who is at actual or potential risk.

What if I think that a crime has occurred?
Adult protective services agencies refer cases to law enforcement if staff
members believe that a crime has occurred. In addition, state law or
federal law may require that you file a report with law enforcement or
other agencies.

What can happen if I do not make a report?
A mandatory reporter's failure to report suspected elder abuse may be
a criminal offense under some state or federal laws. Most importantly,
delaying or failing to report may cause further harm to the older
adult, jeopardize the safety of others, or result in other serious
consequences.

*What if my supervisor disagrees with my assessment and tells me it's not
my responsibility to report? Can this be held against me during
performance reviews?*
Every nurse has an individual responsibility to report suspected cases of
elder abuse. Moreover, mandatory reporters are protected from
retribution as long as the report was made in good faith. It is not
necessary to discuss the report with anyone other than the adult
protective services person who receives the information.

Am I violating confidentiality by making a report?
Reporting laws take precedence over confidentiality standards, including HIPAA requirements.

FIGURE 6.1 APS process for addressing alleged elder abuse.

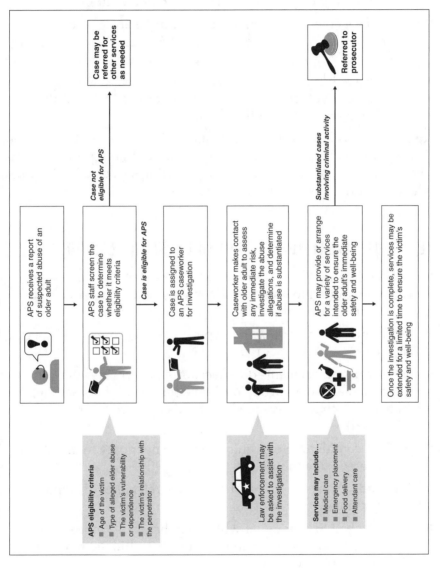

Source: GAO analysis of survey results and interviews from site visits.

131

resources are continually expanding. The following national organizations provide links to these resources:

- Eldercare Locator, www.eldercare.gov: an easy-to-use resource to quicky find contact information for reporting suspected cases according to the zip code in which the older adult lives.

- National Center on Elder Abuse, www.ncea.aoa.gov: click on "Report Elder Abuse," then "Get the Numbers in Your State" to find lists of helplines, hotlines, and referral resources.

- National Adult Protective Services Association, www.napsa-now .org: click "Get Help" to find contact information for adult protective services and other resources.

Appendix A lists contacts for each state related to reporting of elder abuse, with many of these sites providing online reporting forms. Chapter 4 addresses issues related to reporting suspected elder abuse when it occurs in long-term care facilities.

KEY POINTS: WHAT NURSES NEED TO KNOW AND CAN DO

- Nurses in all settings are required to report elder abuse—they are not required to *know* that elder abuse exists but simply to *suspect* its existence.

- State and federal laws define types, covered groups, and specific agencies to receive reports.

- Reporting requirements differ according to whether the suspected abuse occurred in a home setting, a group setting, or a facility that received federal funds (e.g., Medicare, Medicaid).

- HIPAA confidentiality requirements do not apply to mandatory reporting of elder abuse.

- Appendix A lists contacts for each state related to the reporting of elder abuse.

- Nurses need to be familiar with the policies and procedures related to reporting elder abuse in the institution(s) in which they are employed.

REFERENCES

Anetzberger, G. J. (2004). *Philosophy and principles of adult protective services*. Ohio Adult Protective Services Core Curriculum, Ohio Department of Job and Family Services, Columbus, OH.

Campanelli, R. M. (2004). *Letter to Joyce Young HIPAA Government Information Value Exchange for States (GIVES) clarifying enforcement of the Privacy Rule*. Retrieved from www.centeronelderabuse.org/docs/HIPAAGIVES.pdf.

Code of Federal Regulations. (2010). *Title 45: Public Welfare, section 164.512, Uses and disclosures for which an authorization or opportunity to agree or object are not required*. Washington, DC: Government Printing Office.

Frolik, L. A., & Kaplan, R. L. (2014). *Elder law in a nutshell* (6th ed.). St. Paul, MN: West Academic Publishing.

Jirik, S., & Sanders, S. (2014). Analysis of elder abuse statutes across the United States, 2011–2012. *Journal of Gerontological Social Work, 57*, 478–497.

National Adult Protective Services Organization. (n.d.). What is adult protective services? Available at www.napsa-now.org.

Quinn, M. J., & Tomita, S. K. (1986). *Elder abuse and neglect: Causes, diagnosis, and intervention strategies*. New York, NY: Springer Publishing Company.

Schmeidel, A. N., Daly, J. M., Rosenbaum, M. E., Schmuch, G. A., & Jogerst, G. J. (2012). Health care professionals' perspectives on barriers to elder abuse detection and reporting in primary care settings. *Journal of Elder Abuse & Neglect, 24*, 17–36.

Teaster, P. B., Wangmo, T., & Anetzberger, G. J. (2010). A glass half full: The dubious history of elder abuse policy. *Journal of Elder Abuse & Neglect, 22*, 6–15.

7

TOOLS AND GUIDES FOR NURSES TO DETECT ELDER ABUSE

Nursing assessments routinely involve the collection of both subjective and objective data, which are obtained by asking questions and making astute observations. A unique feature of nursing assessment for elder abuse, however, is that subjective data are not readily obtained and objective data can easily be attributed to conditions other than elder abuse. When older adults are in a health care setting, this may be the first—and sometimes only—opportunity they have for talking about an abusive situation they are experiencing or have experienced. Because nurses are the health care professionals who spend the most time with patients in health care settings, they are well positioned to identify indicators of elder abuse.

Because elder abuse is often unrecognized by victims and observers and concealed by victims and perpetrators, nurses may need to approach the situation as detectives rather than assuming that usual assessment strategies will be effective. The process of identifying indicators is complex and includes the following elements: (a) being aware of the possibility that any older adult may be a victim of abuse, (b) recognizing subjective and objective indicators of possible abuse, (c) communicating effectively to elicit details underlying the "red flags," and (d) putting the pieces of the puzzle together to suspect that elder abuse is an actual or potential concern. Elder abuse situations can occur as one-time events or, as is more often the case, they progress gradually. This chapter focuses on the roles of nurses in detecting subtle or gradually progressing cases, because the most blatant cases are more readily identified and usually are being addressed by adult protective services and law enforcement agencies. Roles of nurses in addressing elder abuse in clinical settings are discussed in the chapters found in Parts III and IV.

An additional focus of this chapter is the detection of risks in the broader caregiving situations that are likely to progress to an abusive situation. Nurses are not required to report these at-risk situations, but they can prevent the situations from escalating into reportable conditions or progressing into more serious consequences, as the case in Chapter 14 illustrates. Even when abuse has already occurred, nurses have opportunities to address the consequences and, at a minimum, provide emotional support for victims of elder abuse.

RECOGNIZING INDICATORS OF ABUSE IN OLDER ADULTS

Health care professionals may be reluctant to explore an older adult's experiences with actual or potential abuse for reasons such as lack of time, desire to avoid appearing judgmental, lack of knowledge about what to do, desire to avoid getting involved with family relationships, and questions about whether the situation meets the criteria stated in the law. Cultural factors, as discussed in Chapter 5, also can influence health care professionals' perceptions of elder abuse and their comfort levels with making reports or addressing these issues. One way to overcome these barriers is to recognize that identifying indicators of elder abuse is not time-consuming because most can be identified during the usual nursing assessments of older adults. Another way to overcome these barriers is to remind oneself of the many ways in which nursing interventions can change outcomes and prevent serious consequences—but this can be accomplished only after the situation is identified as abusive or potentially abusive.

It is also important to recognize that no one health care professional is expected to fix or resolve all situations of abuse, but all professionals are expected to provide time for older adults to tell their stories; simply validating their experience can help them move toward solutions (Pisani & Walsh, 2012). The American Nurses Association emphasizes the responsibility of nurses to "safeguard elders from abuse, neglect, and maltreatment" in the *Scope and Standards of Practice* (2004), the *Scope and Standards for Gerontological Nursing Practice* (2001b), and the *Code of Ethics for Nurses With Interpretative Statements* (2001a). In addition, routine assessment of patients for signs and symptoms of abuse is recommended by the Centers for Medicare & Medicaid, The Joint Commission, and the National Gerontological Nursing Association.

As with all nursing assessments, subjective indicators are identified by asking questions and opening the conversation with older adults and others who may have pertinent information. Screening questions can be used to open the conversation about abusive situations and to "normalize" discussion of a difficult topic. Health care institutions often use a simple question such as "Do you feel safe at home?" to screen for domestic violence. This broad type of screening question may elicit information from victims of domestic violence who are unsafe in their homes, but it is rarely effective for opening communication about actual or potential elder abuse situations.

Because of the complexity of elder abuse situations, screening questions need to cover different types, as delineated in the Recognizing Abuse Tool in Box 7.1. This evidence-based tool was developed by the Benjamin Rose Institute on Aging and has been used in the state of Ohio. Focus group members who tested this tool, including nurses, suggested that an initial general question about anyone causing "harm, suffering, or loss" would provide an opener for discussing elder abuse (Ejaz, Bukach, Conway, & Anetzberger, 2014). Nurses in all settings can ask this type of general question and probe further whenever an older adult offers clues to being in an abusive situation. If nurses routinely asked a question such as "On a scale of 1 to 10, how safe do you feel at home?" they would more frequently identify abusive or potentially abusive situations.

When older adults are in health care settings, this may be the first time they recognize the seriousness of their situation and feel safe to talk about it. Thus, it is important to listen for statements that may be a veiled call for help or a "red flag" to a potentially abusive situation. For example, an older adult may give a clue to abusive behavior with a statement such as "He's so stressed at work, he can't help but lose his temper when he comes over to help me."

Objective indicators are identified through physical examinations, laboratory and radiology results, and other commonly used assessment and diagnostic procedures. The types of abuse that are most readily identified through objective measures during usual health assessment procedures are neglect, self-neglect, and all aspects of physical abuse, including sexual abuse. Objective indicators can open communication for more specific questions, such as "How did you get these bruises?" Nursing responsibilities with regard to assessing these types of abuse are discussed in Chapters 10 (neglect, self-neglect, and physical abuse)

BOX 7.1 Recognizing Abuse Tool

Overview

Each section delineates a general question about a form of abuse, followed by examples and possible signs that can be observed during the assessment. If the answer to any question is affirmative, additional questions are asked. Clinical judgment should be used because the information in the tool is not exhaustive.

General Question: Has anyone recently caused you harm, suffering, or loss?

Physical Abuse: Has anyone recently physically harmed you?

Examples

• Hit, pushed, kicked, scratched, strangled, restrained, burned, pulled hair
• Had objects thrown at him or her, such as a book or plate
• Threatened with a knife, gun, or other weapon

Possible signs

• Bruises, welts, cuts, wounds, cigarette or rope burn marks, blood on person/clothes
• Internal injuries, broken or fractured bones, sprains, muscle injuries
• Painful body movements not illness-related, such as limping or trouble with sitting or standing

Sexual Abuse: Has anyone recently sexually harmed you?

Examples

• Raped, sexually assaulted, sexually exploited, molested, hurt or touched without consent
• Intimidated or harassed by sexual innuendos, advances, or threats

(continued)

BOX 7.1 Recognizing Abuse Tool *(continued)*

Possible signs

- Sexually transmitted diseases, vaginal infections, anal bleeding, bruising around the breasts or genital areas, human bite marks, torn or bloodied undergarments
- Coded, vague, or indirect references to sexual assault or unwanted advances
- Feeling afraid or scared of people in positions of power and authority

Psychological or Emotional Abuse: Has anyone recently psychologically harmed you?

Examples

- Yelled at, called names, threatened, harassed, coerced, humiliated
- Stalked or followed around
- Denied/provided insufficient social contact, isolated, locked in a room

Possible signs

- Sense of hopelessness with vague references to mistreatment, passive, helpless, withdrawn
- Anxious, trembling, clinging, fearful, scared of someone/something
- Self-blame for current situation and partner/caregiver behavior

Neglect by Others or Self: Has anyone recently neglected you?

Examples

- Lack of adequate care, such as proper shelter, nutrition, clothing, medication, or transportation
- Lack of adequate supervision, especially in cases of physically or mentally impaired persons
- Lack of treatment for physical health problems
- Extreme hoarding

(continued)

BOX 7.1 Recognizing Abuse Tool *(continued)*

Possible signs

- Unclean physical appearance, inadequately dressed for the weather
- Inadequate living conditions including lack of heat, water, electricity, toilet facilities, food, or supplies in household; unsafe or dirty environment, including insect infestation, unmaintained animals, or presence of fire hazards
- Underweight, physically frail or weak, dehydrated, depressed
- Underuse, overuse, or confusion about prescription or over-the-counter medications

Exploitation: Has anyone recently exploited you financially or otherwise?

Examples

- Property or other assets used, taken, sold, or transferred without consent
- Money withdrawn from bank accounts without knowledge
- Signature forged on checks or other financial or legal documents
- Taking advantage of a relationship for personal benefit or gain

Possible signs

- Overpayment for goods or services, unpaid bills or utilities
- Unexplained changes in power of attorney, wills, or other legal documents
- Missing checks or money, unexplained decreases in bank accounts, missing personal belongings
- Buying expensive gifts for a new friend or significant other

Adapted from Ejaz et al. (2014). Used with permission of Farida K. Ejaz, Benjamin Rose Institute on Aging, Cleveland, OH.

and 16 (sexual abuse). Nurses are less directly involved with identifying indicators of financial exploitation, but this topic is discussed in Chapter 15. Health care professionals can be aware of indicators of psychological abuse, which often occurs in conjunction with other types, when they observe interactions between older adults and their caregivers. The Recognizing Abuse Tool in Box 7.1 identifies possible signs of five types of abuse.

Considerations Related to Elder Abuse in Older Adults With Dementia

Identifying elder abuse in older adults who have dementia is not only challenging but also essential because of their increased vulnerability to all types of abuse in all settings. As with other conditions commonly associated with elder abuse situations, cognitive impairments need to be evaluated in light of the person's decision-making capacity. It is important to recognize that although cognitive impairment increases the risk for elder abuse, the diagnosis of dementia does not necessarily indicate that the person is unable to make or be involved with decisions about the care he or she receives, the relationships he or she desires, or any other aspect of his or her life. Also, dementia does not necessarily interfere with the person's ability to talk reliably about abuse he or she is experiencing or has experienced. This is particularly true during early and middle stages of dementia. Another important consideration is that even if cognitive impairments or communication barriers affect the ability of older adults to discuss or report their abusive situations, nurses can observe indicators of elder abuse. The signs of five types of abuse delineated in the Recognizing Abuse Tool (Box 7.1) and clues to elder abuse in the broader caregiver situation (discussed in the next section) are applicable to all older adults regardless of their cognitive function.

COMMUNICATING WITH OLDER ADULTS TO ELICIT INFORMATION

In addition to being aware of clues to elder abuse, it is important to be aware of reasons that elder abuse victims may be reluctant to talk about their situation, particularly when they depend on a caregiver who is responsible for the abusive situation. Some reasons that older adults may not disclose their situation are as follows:

- Lack of insight about or awareness of their own situation
- Inability to report details, due to cognitive impairment, emotional limitations, physical disability, or disorders that affect communication
- Love and protection of the perpetrator
- Feelings of responsibility toward the perpetrator/caregiver
- Feelings of shame, embarrassment, self-blame

- Fear of retaliation by perpetrator
- Fear of alternative arrangement (e.g., moving to an institutional setting, caregiver abandonment)
- Poor self-esteem, feeling that the abuse is deserved
- Mistrust of outsiders

One step toward overcoming these barriers is to be perceived by older adults as a trusted professional who accepts them and their situation without judgment and has a genuine desire to help. In addition, older adults must have confidence that talking to the nurse will not worsen their situation or result in an undesirable change. Despite the barriers to and precautions about revealing evidence of elder abuse, older adults are likely to disclose their experiences if a trusted and caring professional asks nonthreatening questions in a setting where they feel respected and are assured of privacy and confidentiality.

Obtaining privacy is often the first challenge in talking with older adults to "hear their story" when family members or other caregivers who are responsible for an abusive situation insist on being present. Even though "hovering" behaviors of family or caregivers are not necessarily a clue to elder abuse, nurses need to create opportunities for one-on-one private discussions with older adults. When others insist on being present, nurses can use strategies such as the following ones:

- Say to the older adult: "I understand that you might want your son here while we talk, but it's important that I have a chance to talk with you alone so I can hear from you about how you are managing."
- Say to the family or caregiver: "I want to hear from you about how your mother manages, but first I need time to talk with her alone so I can hear her perspective."
- Arrange for another team member, such as a social worker, to meet with family or caregivers in another room while the nurse talks with the older adult in private.

Box 7.2 describes strategies for communicating with older adults to elicit information about abusive or potentially abusive situations.

RECOGNIZING INDICATORS OF AND RISKS FOR ABUSE IN THE BROADER CAREGIVING SITUATION

In addition to being aware of indicators and risks in older adults themselves, nurses need to be aware of indicators and risks in the

BOX 7.2 Strategies for Communicating With Older Adults to Identify Their Abusive or Potentially Abusive Situations

Guidelines for verbal and nonverbal communication

• Express empathic concern
• Communicate that client's feelings are important
• Do not communicate judgment about the alleged abuser
• Do not minimize or dismiss an older adult's reports or feelings based on cognitive impairment, a history of paranoia, or any other reason
• Ask how you can obtain more details from someone else but do not communicate that you question the validity of what the person reports
• Communicate a sense of hope
• Provide assurance that health care professionals will respect the older adult's right to make his or her own decisions, as long as the person has not been judged incompetent by a court

What to say

• "I appreciate that you're willing to talk about this."
• "I will do my best to help you without jeopardizing your relationship with your caregivers."
• "Can you give me an example of how your nephew mistreats you?"
• "I'm sorry that you are being treated that way."
• "It must be very difficult to be in the situation you're in."
• "Perhaps we can find ways to address what you call his 'temper tantrums' that would be beneficial to both of you."

What *not* to say

• "That's shocking."
• "It's hard to believe that your son would do that to you."
• "We'll make sure that things change."
• "He sounds like he's a real scumbag [or any other judgmental description]."
• "It's unfortunate that you have to depend on your granddaughter for help."
• "I'm obligated to report this, but don't worry, the adult protective services agency will get to the bottom of this and your nephew will get what he deserves."

(continued)

BOX 7.2 Strategies for Communicating With Older Adults to Identify Their Abusive or Potentially Abusive Situations *(continued)*

- "Even though you want to stay in your own home, you'd get much better care in a nursing home."

Questions to ask in one-on-one conversations with an older adult

- "Have you been hit, smacked, or in any other way physically mistreated by anyone who currently provides care for you?"

- "Have you ever felt neglected or ignored by anyone who provides care for you?"

- "Can you describe any times when you felt your needs were not met by someone whom you expected to care for you?"

- "Has anyone yelled or screamed at you or said anything that felt threatening, for example, told you that you would be put in a nursing home?"

- "How would you describe your nephew's personality when he is caring for you?"

- "What is the most difficult aspect of having the outside caregivers come into your house?"

- "Do you have any concerns about your safety or your belongings when the caregivers are in your house?"

- "Have you had (or do you have) questions about how your finances are managed or about your assets?"

- "Have you signed legal papers that you have questions about or don't agree with?"

- "Has anyone forced you to do things that you didn't want to do?"

broader caregiving situations. For example, when nurses work with family members and unpaid or informal caregivers who provide care for dependent older adults, they have many opportunities to detect clues to domestic elder abuse. Nurses who make home visits have direct opportunities to identify risks not only in the interactions between older adults and their caregivers but also in the physical environment. For instance, nurses can observe whether the basic necessities, such as food, medicine, or clothing, are adequately provided for the older adult.

Because many situations of elder abuse involve paid or unpaid caregivers of dependent older adults, elder abuse scholars have focused on identifying risks for or indicators of domestic elder abuse in the relationships between the caregiver and the older adult. Chapter 14 illustrates application of a Risk of Abuse Tool to an unfolding case, with emphasis on the roles of nurses in addressing at-risk situations of domestic elder abuse. The Alleged Abuser Scale (Box 7.3) is an evidence-based tool delineating indicators of possible elder abuse that would be observed in a trusted other.

COMMUNICATING WITH CAREGIVERS WHO ARE POSSIBLE ABUSERS

Health care settings can provide safe opportunities not only for older adults to disclose situations of elder abuse, but also for family and caregivers to acknowledge the need for help with stressful situations. Although many perpetrators of elder abuse are strongly motivated to avoid disclosure of the situation, it is important to recognize that some caregivers who are abusive, or at risk of becoming so, may be willing to talk about their situation and accept help if they feel they will not be judged or punished. It is also important to recognize that sometimes elder abuse is unintentional and may even be unrecognized by older adults and others involved with the situation. These situations, as well as other at-risk situations, are often amenable to relatively simple nursing interventions. For example, when family caregivers are abusive because they lack the skills or knowledge to provide appropriate care, nurses can teach and role model care techniques and initiate referrals for ongoing support and help with development of caregiving skills. Caregivers are likely to open up and discuss difficult situations if they view the nurse as an empathic and trusted professional who will help resolve problems and reduce stress. Box 7.4 can be used as a guide to elicit details that provide clues to abusive or potentially abusive situations.

PUTTING THE PIECES OF THE PUZZLE TOGETHER

Nurses can use tools and guides to identify indicators of and risks for abuse, but they also need to go a step further and put the assessment pieces together to determine whether a situation meets the requirements for reporting or indicates the need for interventions. Because most health care providers have only short-term or intermittent contact with an older adult, it is imperative that each and every health care

BOX 7.3 Observations About a Suspected Abuser

Observations about the suspected abuser who is responsible for care
The individual . . .

. . . blames others for his or her problems

. . . has had a conflictive relationship with the older adult

. . . gives improbable or contradictory explanations about the health or injuries of the older adult

. . . seems to lack necessary skills or knowledge to provide appropriate care

. . . seems to have difficulty resolving stressful or difficult situations

. . . exhibits behavioral problems, such as being disruptive or aggressive

. . . is critical, suspicious, and/or cautious with professionals

. . . has mental health problems (e.g., depression, obsession, phobias)

. . . has problems with family relationships

. . . is reluctant to accept help

Observations related to the relationship with the older adult
There are signs that the individual . . .

. . . makes it difficult for professionals to talk alone with the older adult

. . . displays an attitude of indifference toward the older adult

. . . views the care of the older adult as an unwelcome burden

. . . insults the older adult

. . . forces the older adult to act against his or her own will

. . . assaults the older adult

. . . threatens the older adult

. . . does not allow the older adult to interact with other people

. . . does not allow the older adult to make decisions or manage money, even though the person is capable of doing so

. . . unnecessarily limits the older adult's activities

Touza, Prado, and Segura (2012). Adapted with permission of The Haworth Maltreatment & Trauma Press via Copyright Clearance Center. (Taylor & Francis Ltd, http://www.tandfonline.com).

BOX 7.4 Strategies for Communicating With Caregivers Who Are Suspected or Potential Abusers

Guidelines for verbal and nonverbal communication

- Express empathy
- Validate that the caregiver's concerns are important
- Elicit information about stresses of caregiving
- Communicate a nonjudgmental attitude

Ask general questions about caregiving

- "Can you describe a typical day, beginning with when you and your husband awaken and ending with when you go to bed?"
- "Do you have caregiving responsibilities during the night?"
- "What are the things you do for your wife on a daily basis? . . . on a weekly basis?—less frequently (e.g., haircuts, medical appointments, holidays)?"
- "What are the most difficult aspects of meeting your father's needs?"
- "How would you describe your mother's personality and behaviors during the past few months?"
- "Your situation sounds very stressful. How is it for you to be in the position you are in?"
- "How do you cope with this difficult situation?"
- "What supports do you have for providing care?"
- "What responsibilities outside the home do you have?"
- "Do you have time for activities that you personally enjoy or find enriching?"

Ask questions related to possible indicators of elder abuse

- Bruising, wounds, evidence of physical abuse: "Can you tell me how your mother got those bruises on her arms and chest?"
- Neglect or unreasonable delay in seeking care: "I'm wondering why your father didn't see his doctor in the past months while his symptoms were worsening. Can you give me any insight into this?"
- Weight loss, laboratory indicators of malnutrition, dehydration: "There are indications that your grandmother has not been eating and drinking enough. Can you tell me about problems she is having with this?"
- Observations or reports of aggressive behaviors: "I know it's challenging to care for someone who frequently hits those who provide care. When this happens, how do you handle the situation? Do his behaviors ever cause you to lose your temper or yell at him?"

provider makes astute observations and documents these observations in the patient's medical record. In addition, nurses can discuss their observations with other members of the health care team and professionally share concerns about risks for or indicators of elder abuse.

Tools such as the ones delineated in this chapter and those that are incorporated in policies and procedures where nurses are employed provide a basic guide for raising suspicions about abusive or potentially abusive situations. However, these indicators are not unique to abusive situations and alternative explanations can be given to explain their occurrence. For example, older adults often experience bruises and fractures even in the most supportive settings or primarily due to age-associated conditions. Thus, health care professionals are challenged not only to be detectives with regard to identifying indicators but also to draw on professional intuitive skills to develop their awareness of abusive or potentially abusive situations. In addition, like other clinically complicated conditions, elder abuse situations require that all health care professionals communicate with other team members about their assessments so plans can be developed to resolve problems. Perhaps the most challenging aspect of detecting clues to an abusive situation is taking the next step to address the situation. Although nurses have a legal responsibility to report suspected cases, they have many roles in addressing actual, suspected, and at-risk elder abuse situations in clinical settings. In addition, they have essential roles within the context of a team of other health care professionals and a network of community-based services. These roles are discussed in Part III and illustrated in cases in Part IV.

KEY POINTS: WHAT NURSES NEED TO KNOW AND CAN DO

- Subjective and objective indicators of elder abuse can be identified during usual nursing assessments and through the use of screening tools, such as the one delineated in Box 7.1.

- Nurses can use communication strategies to elicit information about abusive or potentially abusive situations (Boxes 7.2 and 7.4).

- Nurses have essential roles in observing for indicators of actual or potential abuse in the broader caregiving situation (Box 7.3).

- Nurses need to be familiar with policies and procedures related to screening for elder abuse in the institution(s) in which they work.

■ In addition to using tools and assessment guides, it is imperative to apply intuitive nursing skills to put the puzzle pieces together.

REFERENCES

American Nurses Association. (2001a). *Code of ethics for nurses with interpretative statements.* Silver Spring, MD: Author.

American Nurses Association. (2001b). *Scope and standards for gerontological nursing practice.* Silver Spring, MD: Author.

American Nurses Association. (2004). *Scope and standards of practice.* Silver Spring, MD: Author.

Ejaz, F. K., Bukach, A. M., Conway, A. K., & Anetzberger, G. (2014). *Development of online training modules on abuse, neglect, and exploitation for care managers in MyCare Ohio.* Report to the Ohio Department of Aging and the Administration for Community Living.

Pisani, L. D., & Walsh, C. A. (2012). Screening for elder abuse in hospitalized older adults with dementia. *Journal of Elder Abuse & Neglect, 24,* 195–215.

Touza, C., Prado, C., & Segura, M. (2012). Detection scales for the risk of domestic abuse and self-negligent behavior in elderly persons (EDMA). *Journal of Elder Abuse & Neglect, 24,* 312–325.

8

ETHICAL ISSUES RELATED TO ELDER ABUSE FOR NURSES

Laws can define elder abuse and tools can facilitate the identification of indicators of abuse; however, these laws and tools cannot answer all the questions that arise when nurses care for older adults who are in situations of actual or potential abuse. These questions begin when signs of elder abuse are imprecise, as is often the case, and they end only after the nurse is no longer providing care for the older adult. Even then, nurses often are troubled by the "what ifs" of decisions that they made and actions that they did or did not take. In a society that highly values autonomy and self-determination (i.e., each individual has an inherent right to personal choices and decisions), an overriding question in most situations of elder abuse is: "To what extent is this person knowingly choosing his or her situation?" This question is not easy to answer, but it is at the crux of ethical issues that are addressed by health care professionals.

Nurses usually do not have a leading role in addressing ethical concerns, but they always have crucial professional responsibilities—and major supporting roles—with regard to identifying and resolving these important aspects of patient care. This chapter provides an overview of ethical issues related to elder abuse situations that are often addressed in health care settings. In addition, it provides information about professional resources that nurses can draw on and personal strategies they can use to become more comfortable when they address ethical issues related to elder abuse. Case examples illustrate strategies that nurses can use to help resolve ethical dilemmas associated with elder abuse situations.

ISSUES RELATED TO DECISION-MAKING CAPACITY

Nurses are routinely involved with obtaining a patient's informed consent for all types of health-related procedures, and sometimes this responsibility requires professional judgment about the patient's decision-making capacity. In general, professionals judge a patient's ability to provide informed consent according to questions such as the following:

- Does the individual understand the facts of the situation?
- Does the individual understand the risks and benefits of different options?
- Does the individual express a free choice about his or her situation?

When answers to questions such as these are not clear, health care professionals follow their institutional policies and procedures to ascertain the patient's ability to provide informed consent. Many times, they can also rely on a legally designated health care proxy who is clearly acting in the patient's best interests.

In elder abuse situations, nurses have similar responsibilities related to informed consent, but the issues are usually broader, more complex, and ill defined. For example, the following questions are often addressed as an integral aspect of discharge plans:

- What is the best interests of the older adult?
- What alternatives are realistic within the limits of the situation?
- To what extent does the older adult have the right to refuse services when risks to safety are involved?

Questions also arise about whether other individuals involved with decision making are acting in the best interests of the older adult, or whether they are attempting to enforce decisions that conflict with the wishes and best interests of the older adult. Sometimes these individuals have legal authority to represent the older adult, but many times they exert control over the situation primarily through their relationship with the older person. Even when the individuals have legal authority to make decisions, they may not be acting in the best interests of the older adult. These types of situations can present ethical dilemmas for nurses who are providing the care.

Legal Aspects of Consent, Decision-Making Capacity, and Undue Influence

Health care professionals are usually concerned about decision-making capacity in relation to issues such as medical or surgical interventions, basic care needs, and risks to safety. In elder abuse situations, the focus of decision-making capacity can include broader issues, such as protection of one's assets (financial abuse), protecting oneself from verbal or emotional abuse (psychological abuse), and consent to participate in intimate relationships (sexual abuse). Legal aspects of consent, decision-making capacity, and undue influence are defined in laws, but these definitions are not necessarily specific to elder abuse. Box 8.1 summarizes information about these legal terms in relation to many types of elder abuse. The American Bar Association (2014) developed these as a guide for law enforcement officers in the United States, but application of these descriptions varies according to state laws.

Clinical Aspects of Decision-Making Capacity

When health care professionals are called upon to determine a patient's decision-making capacity, the assessment process is complex and challenging for reasons such as:

- All the following should be considered in relation to decision-making capacity: mental status; physical, mental, and emotional health; usual lifestyle, philosophy of life, past capacity to make decisions, and history of interpersonal relationships.
- Indicators are often "gray" rather than "black and white."
- Mental status and other variables can fluctuate considerably, both short-term and long-term.
- Personal decisions are not necessarily based on logic and deliberation and are strongly influenced by factors such as values, emotions, culture, experiences, religious beliefs, and resources.
- Other people exert varying degrees of influence over one's decisions and it is difficult to assess the effects and extent of these influences.
- Personal decisions directly affect one's quality of life, which is defined uniquely by each individual.

Elder abuse situations often involve family, friends, caregivers, and other individuals who are part of the problem but may also need

BOX 8.1 Legal Terms Associated With Elder Abuse

Consent

- Definition: a decision to do something or to allow something to happen, for example, giving informed consent to have a medical procedure.
- May be given in writing, verbally, or through behavioral indicators such as nodding. The nature of the decision determines what method of demonstrating consent is necessary.
- To give legally valid consent, a person must (a) have decision-making capacity, (b) be knowledgeable about the true nature of an act, and (c) act freely and voluntarily.
- Reasons for the inability to provide consent may include lack of decision-making capacity or fraud and misrepresentations about the real circumstances of a transaction.

Decision-Making Capacity

- Definition: the cognitive ability to make a decision.
- The law presumes that adults have capacity, unless a court decides differently and appoints a guardian or conservator to make decisions for the adult.
- Capacity is usually not black or white, all or nothing. It may fluctuate over time and even over the course of a day. For example, capacity is likely to fluctuate during the day in people with Alzheimer's disease and other types of progressive dementia.
- Just because a person is old or has an illness or condition that affects cognitive abilities does not mean the person lacks capacity. For example, a person in the early to middle stages of Alzheimer's disease may have capacity to make some or all decisions.
- Some of the conditions that affect capacity are disease, disability, alcohol, drugs, and nutrition.
- Legally, different standards of capacity apply to different types of decisions. For example, complex decisions usually require a higher standard of capacity, but for financial matters, the minimal standard is that a person must understand the nature of the decision being made and the actual or potential effect of that decision.

(continued)

BOX 8.1 Legal Terms Associated With Elder Abuse *(continued)*

Undue Influence

- Definition: the use of power in a relationship to exploit another person's trust, fear, and dependency.
- State courts define undue influence differently but they generally look at the following: (a) relationship between the alleged influencer and alleged victim (e.g., family, care provider, financial advisor, attorney); (b) the alleged victim's vulnerability to undue influence (e.g., associated with grief, illness, cognitive impairment, medications); (c) the alleged influencer's opportunity to gain control, for example, by socially isolating the alleged victim; (d) whether the alleged victim's decisions were the outcome of the undue influence (e.g., were they made suddenly, were they inconsistent with previous decisions, or did the alleged influencer choose the lawyer and sit in on all the meetings with the lawyer?).
- A person who has decision-making capacity can be unduly influenced, but it is easier to commit undue influence on someone who has diminished capacity.
- Generally, a victim of undue influence will not recognize what is happening and will side with the perpetrator.

Relevance to Elder Abuse

The legal concepts of consent, decision-making capacity, and undue influence—or some combination of them—are critical issues in many cases of elder abuse. These concepts are relevant in the following ways:

- Present decisions: for example, can the alleged victim agree to or refuse to accept help or services?
- Past decisions: for example, did the alleged victim have the capacity to deed his property or sign his or her will knowingly and voluntarily, or was it really the result of undue influence?
- If an alleged victim lacks decision-making capacity, a court-appointed guardian or conservator may be necessary to protect the person from harm.

Source: Consent, Decision-Making Capacity, and Undue Influence, from American Bar Association (2014). Adapted with permission. All rights reserved. This information or any or portion thereof may not be copied or disseminated in any form or by any means or stored in an electronic database or retrieval system without the express written consent of the American Bar Association.

to be part of the solutions. Another consideration is that a person's decision-making capacity in a domestic elder abuse situation may be compromised by factors such as a desire to protect a caregiver from prosecution or a feeling of responsibility for adult children who are financially dependent or substance abusers.

Under all circumstances, certain principles apply. One basic principle is that conclusions should not be based solely on a person's age or diagnosis. For example, a diagnosis of dementia or an age of more than 85 years does not automatically affect one's decision-making capacity. Another principle is that decision making is not an "all or nothing" process and is affected by many variables, such as the complexity of the decision and the person's prior level of understanding and knowledge about the decision. As an example, a person with dementia may be able to decide about the appointment of a surrogate decision maker but may not be able to participate in a complex decision about medical treatment options for cancer. Cultural factors also play an important role in decision making, as discussed in Chapter 5.

In clinical settings, assessment of decision-making capacity is a complex process in which information is shared among patients, practitioners, and family and others who are involved with the care and affected by the outcomes. A characteristic of many domestic elder abuse cases, however, is that health care professionals need to also assess the actions, abilities, and intentions of family and caregivers to determine the appropriateness of involving them. In some situations, practitioners need to purposefully exclude certain so-called concerned parties from discussions. Thus, in elder abuse situations, nurses may need to make ethical decisions about sharing information with families, even in situations in which the family members declare their right to be involved. Whenever nurses have questions about the benefit or risk of sharing information, they need to discuss the situation with other professionals, as these situations require a team approach.

Determination of Competency

It is important to recognize the difference between clinical aspects of decision-making capacity and determination of competency, because these terms are pertinent to many elder abuse situations. In contrast to decision-making capacity, which applies to specific circumstances, competency is a legal term that refers to one's overall abilities to fulfill one's role and handle one's affairs in a responsible manner. All adults (usually defined as age 18 years) are presumed to be competent and able to participate in legally binding decisions. Although state laws differ in their definitions and specific provisions, in general this legal right extends to decisions related to health care and living conditions, even including decisions that involve major personal risks.

In health care settings, legally appointed surrogate decision makers (e.g., those with durable power of attorney) can make decisions about health care for adults who lack decision-making capacity. This arrangement works well when an acceptable and appropriate plan of care can be developed and agreed upon by all involved, including health care professionals, the older adult, and family and caregivers. However, situations of elder abuse often involve barriers to this process such as the following:

- Conflicts exist among the people involved with making and implementing decisions or between the older adult and others.

- Questions are raised about the integrity or ability of any of the decision makers.

- The situation involves risks to safety that cannot be resolved.

- The older adult or others involved are not willing to accept appropriate interventions.

- The older adult's decision-making capacity is questionable and there is no reliable surrogate decision maker.

Circumstances such as these usually indicate the need for adult protective services. Even if the situation is not clearly elder abuse, adult protective services have major roles in working with older adults whose competency and decision-making capacity is questionable. Although nurses in clinical settings are rarely involved with legal processes, they are often in positions of advising families about legal interventions.

State laws define the process for determining competency, which usually includes an extensive evaluation by at least one medical professional, such as a physician or psychiatrist. If the court (e.g., a probate court) determines that the person is incompetent, the judge assigns either a partial or a full guardianship (also called a conservatorship). With a partial guardianship, the incompetent person continues to make limited decisions; with a full guardianship, the person loses all of his or her rights to make decisions. Although additional court action can revoke or reverse a guardianship after it has been granted, the guardianship typically remains in place until the incompetent person dies.

Usually, guardianship is initiated only as a last resort when no other legal intervention is appropriate because it is a drastic measure that takes away rights and entails court proceedings and ongoing court monitoring.

WHAT NURSES NEED TO KNOW ABOUT ADULT PROTECTIVE SERVICES ETHICAL GUIDELINES

For decades, the National Association of Adult Protective Services (NAPSA) has addressed ethical issues related to elder abuse, including concerns about respecting an older adult's right to self-determination versus supporting a plan that includes risks or is not consistent with what health care professionals recommend. The NAPSA guideline for ethical principles describes the "guiding value" as "Every action taken by Adult Protective Services must balance the duty to protect the safety of the vulnerable adult with the adult's right to self-determination" (NAPSA, 2004). Ethical principles that shape adult protective services include the following:

- Adults have the right to be safe.
- Adults retain all their civil and constitutional rights unless some of these rights have been restricted by court action.
- Adults have the right to make decisions that do not conform to societal norms as long as these decisions do not harm others.
- Adults are presumed to have decision-making capacity unless a court adjudicates otherwise.
- Adults have the right to accept or refuse services.

In addition, it is important to know that adult protective services support the least restrictive alternative, even when a more restrictive environment would presumably provide better care. Health care professionals can advise older adults and their decision makers about a plan that is likely to provide better care (e.g., a skilled nursing facility for rehabilitation vs. returning to home), but they cannot mandate that this plan be implemented. Box 8.2 presents a hierarchy of ethical principles for adult protective services.

BOX 8.2 Hierarchy of Principles of Adult Protective Services

1. *Freedom Over Safety:* The older adult has a right to choose to live at risk for harm, providing he or she is capable of making that choice, harms no one, and commits no crime.

2. *Self-Determination:* The older adult has a right to personal choices and decisions until such time that he or she delegates, or the court grants, the responsibility to someone else.

3. *Participation in Decision Making:* The older adult has a right to receive information to make informed choices and to participate in all decisions affecting his or her circumstances to the extent that he or she is able.

4. *Least Restrictive Alternative:* The older adult has a right to service alternatives that maximize choice and minimize lifestyle disruption.

5. *Primacy of the Adult:* The practitioner's primary responsibility is to serve the older adult, not anyone else (e.g., community people concerned about appearances or a family member concerned about finances).

6. *Confidentiality:* The older adult has a right to privacy and confidentiality.

7. *Benefit of Doubt:* If there is evidence that the older adult is making a reasoned choice, the practitioner has a responsibility to assure that the benefit of doubt is in favor of the older adult.

8. *Do No Harm:* The practitioner has a responsibility to take no action that places the older adult at greater risk of harm.

9. *Avoidance of Blame:* The practitioner has a responsibility to understand the origins of any mistreatment and to commit no action that would antagonize the perpetrator and so reduce the chance of terminating the mistreatment.

10. *Maintenance of the Family:* If the perpetrator is a family member, the practitioner has a responsibility to deal with the mistreatment as a family problem and to try to find appropriate services to resolve the problem.

Source: Anetzberger (1982). Reprinted by permission of author.

CASE EXAMPLES OF WHAT NURSES CAN DO TO ADDRESS ETHICAL ISSUES RELATED TO ELDER ABUSE

CASE 8.1 When the Wishes of an Older Adult Conflict With the Plans of the Family Caregiver

Background

Even in the best situations, plans for care of a dependent older adult often require that health care professionals address conflicting needs and wishes of the older adult and family and others who are resources for care. These conflicts arise from many sources, such as competing demands for the caregiver's time, differing expectations of the older adult and the family member, financial concerns related both to the cost of paid caregiving and the loss of income for family caregivers, unacceptability or unavailability of agency-based services, and long distance between the family member and the older adult. Nurses often become aware of conflicting needs and wishes because they provide care for the dependent older adult and also are a primary point of contact for the family. Sometimes these conflicts involve ethical dilemmas related to elder abuse, as in the case of Mrs. Wong and her son.

Clinical Situation

Mrs. Wong was born in China and moved to San Francisco 10 years ago when she was 67 to live with her son and his family after he established a successful business in the United States. Mrs. Wong was admitted to the hospital for a fractured hip 3 days ago. When Nurse Kathleen is preparing Mrs. Wong for discharge, Mrs. Wong confides that she does not want to return to her son's house because she would have to navigate a flight of steps into the house and another flight to her bedroom and she is afraid she would "feel like a prisoner and never get out once I'm in their house again." She also states that even though her son says she tripped when going downstairs, she thinks he pushed her because he was behind her and in a hurry to get downstairs. She knows she is eligible for skilled rehabilitation but she tells the nurse, "My son says if I don't go back to his house he will send me back to China to live with my younger son. Besides, in our family the oldest son makes all the decisions about his parents so you need to talk with him about discharge plans. If he tells you I am going back to his house, that's what

(continued)

CASE 8.1 When the Wishes of an Older Adult Conflict With the Plans of the Family Caregiver *(continued)*

will happen." Mrs. Wong tearfully confides that she wanted to move to the assisted living facility that recently opened specifically for Chinese Americans, but her son would not let her use her money for that.

Nursing assessments document that Mrs. Wong was delusional and disoriented for 24 hours postoperatively. Two days ago, Mrs. Wong's son told Nurse Kathleen that his mother had been diagnosed with dementia and "you can never believe a word she says." He also told the nurse that he had helped his mother down the stairs and then she fell at the bottom when her knees buckled. He added, "It's no wonder that she broke her hip because she's supposed to take calcium for osteoporosis but I find the pills in the wastebasket because she says she has a hard time swallowing them."

What Nurse Kathleen Thinks

I don't know if Mrs. Wong's concerns about discharge are valid. According to her son, she has dementia but that's not documented on her chart. I don't know what she was like before surgery, but her mental status was certainly altered when I took care of her after surgery. Today she seems to know what she's talking about but she probably just wants to blame her son because she fell down the stairs and fractured her hip. On the other hand, Mrs. Wong's son seemed to be pretty stern with her and he made a point of finding me at the nurses' station the other day so he could tell me I shouldn't believe a word she says. Maybe he does have something to hide. Maybe I'm detecting signs of elder abuse, or financial exploitation.

Although I have concerns about this discharge plan, the doctor established it yesterday with Mrs. Wong's son when I was not on duty. I have six other patients to care for and my shift ends in an hour so I don't have time to question a discharge plan that seems reasonable. Based on my concerns and observations, though, I should do something about it.

What Nurse Kathleen Does

Nurse Kathleen documents today's conversation in the electronic medical record and assures that the information will be transmitted to the home care agency that is providing skilled care services.

(continued)

CASE 8.1   When the Wishes of an Older Adult Conflict With the Plans of the Family Caregiver *(continued)*

In addition, the nurse asks the doctor to add a request for skilled social work services on the referral for skilled nursing and physical therapy home care that has already been initiated.

Resolution of Ethical Dilemma

Nurse Kathleen does not have enough information to report the case to adult protective services nor does she believe that a report would resolve the situation, so she communicates pertinent information to the home care agency and relies on the skilled social worker services to follow up.

CASE 8.2   When There Is a Conflict Between Self-Determination and Safety of an Older Adult

Background

Nurses may experience conflicts between their responsibility to protect their patients from harm and their responsibility to honor each person's right to choices and decisions. It is important to recognize that safety is not a paramount goal for many older adults, and should not be the sole criterion for decisions about their living arrangements. When decisions have a major impact on a person's quality of life, questions about safety and risks need to be considered within the context of the person's values and other influencing factors. When older adults value independence over risks, health care providers can facilitate plans that help reduce the risk while at the same time respecting the person's right to self-determination.

Clinical Situation

Mr. Cunningham, a 79-year-old patient admitted for a stroke, no longer requires acute care. In addition to the diagnosis of CVA, his admitting

(continued)

CASE 8.2 When There Is a Conflict Between Self-Determination and Safety of an Older Adult *(continued)*

diagnoses included dehydration, malnutrition, atrial fibrillation, history of multiple falls, and urinary tract infection. He lives with his two dogs in the house he was born in. He is eligible for admission to a nursing home for skilled therapies, but he adamantly refuses to consider any plan that does not include a discharge to home. He tells Nurse Paulette that his daughter is staying at his house and caring for his dogs but he has no one to care for them after she leaves. Mr. Cunningham's daughter, Cindy, will be returning to her own home, 800 miles away, in 3 days. Cindy reported that her father's house was "a shambles when I arrived but I did my best to get rid of the worst of the trash." She also reported that her father's dogs looked "like miserable street animals." Cindy visits about twice a year and has tried to get her father to accept home-delivered meals, housekeeping, and other services, but he has always adamantly refused. Several times Cindy hired a friend's daughter to help address her father's basic needs, but he would never let her in the house. Nurses have described Mr. Cunningham as "feisty and determined" and his daughter describes him as "a loner and curmudgeon who has alienated any friends he ever had." Cindy says she will not challenge his wishes to return home and she respects his right to refuse services, even though the therapists recommend that he be in a supervised setting for his own safety.

What Nurse Paulette Thinks

I have serious concerns about the safety of a plan for him to return to his own home, especially if he refuses any services. Even his daughter said it was a hopeless situation and I should not be bothered. When I reviewed his home-going medications with him, he told me he has no intention of taking "all those new pills you've been forcing on me since I was admitted." Then he closed his eyes and pretended he was asleep so I couldn't continue with our discussion.

What Nurse Paulette Does

Nurse Paulette talks with Cindy in a conference room to discuss the situation. When Cindy confides that "there's a good reason I live in another part of the country and I have no intention of dedicating my

(continued)

CASE 8.2 When There Is a Conflict Between Self-Determination and Safety of an Older Adult *(continued)*

life to him. He never was around for me when I needed him," the nurse communicates an empathetic and nonjudgmental response. Nurse Paulette then explains that Mr. Cunningham's medical diagnoses and history of frequent falls would qualify him for skilled care at home. She further suggests that even though he has refused to consider going to a skilled nursing facility, he may accept skilled care at home, especially if he knows this is covered by his Medicare insurance. When Cindy and Nurse Paulette present this option to Mr. Cunningham, he reluctantly agrees to sign the consent for a referral. On the referral form for home care, the nurse documents the need for in-home evaluations of the patient's safety, risks for falls, and adherence to medications. In addition, Nurse Paulette gives Cindy contact information for the local adult protective services agency and suggests that Cindy can request an investigation if she becomes aware of significant risks after her father is home and no longer receiving home care services.

Resolution of Ethical Dilemma

Based on ethical principles of adult protective services, Nurse Paulette respected Mr. Cunningham's right to freedom over safety but she also tried to minimize the risks. Nurse Paulette used strategies to gain Mr. Cunningham's acceptance of home-based services and she taught Cindy about resources for initiating an investigation if she is concerned about his refusal to accept services in the future.

CASE 8.3 When a Family Member Exerts Undue Control Over Plans for an Older Adult

Background

Domestic elder abuse situations often include elements of psychological abuse arising from an unbalanced or unhealthy controlling relationship between the dependent person and the caregiver. Sometimes the

(continued)

CASE 8.3 When a Family Member Exerts Undue Control Over Plans for an Older Adult *(continued)*

control issues go both ways, for example, when an adult child is dependent on a parent for financial and housing support and the parent is dependent on the adult child for care so he or she can continue living in his or her own home. These situations can be mutually beneficial and are not necessarily abusive. However, these situations may be abusive when they involve undue influence, unfair financial advantage, or unnecessary control over the older adult. Similarly, elements of elder abuse are present when adult children benefit from spreading false information to convince others that the parent is incapable of making independent decisions. The case of Gertrude illustrates the role of a nurse in a community-based setting in addressing a situation involving an ethical responsibility to protect an older adult's rights.

Faith community nurses (also called parish nurses) provide informal services for clients who live in independent settings, often on a regular basis over many months or years. Their roles include assessment, health counseling, referrals for services, and advocacy for clients who are members of their faith based community. Nurse Robert works part-time as a faith-community nurse and provides support services for parishioners who care for dependent family members.

Clinical Situation

When Nurse Robert met Gertrude, he was initially impressed with her charm and social skills, but he also recognized the telltale—albeit subtle—signs of dementia. For example, Gertrude's short-term memory was very poor and she frequently repeated her narrow repertoire of familiar phrases. Gertrude had recently moved in with her daughter, Amelia, and son-in-law. The couple's eight foster children and two adopted children (all toddlers through teens) also lived in the house and were home-schooled. Amelia had previously told Nurse Robert that her mother needed to move in with her because she had dementia and was not receiving proper care.

Before moving in with Amelia, Gertrude had been living in her own home, which she shared with her second-marriage husband of 23 years. Amelia claimed that Gertrude was not legally married because her mother and Homer had been married in Niagara Falls,

(continued)

CASE 8.3 When a Family Member Exerts Undue Control Over Plans for an Older Adult *(continued)*

Canada, and never had a ceremony in the United States. Amelia had started Gertrude on a complicated regimen of nonprescription substances that were marketed as "miracle cures for memory problems." Amelia explained that the regimen was "too complicated for Homer to oversee and too expensive to let my mother be in charge of." In addition, Homer was incapable of cooking healthy meals, so Amelia and her husband generously offered to have Gertrude move in with them. Amelia also reported that Homer was an unsafe driver, so he was not allowed to take her anywhere.

When Nurse Robert met privately with Gertrude, she repeatedly told him that she wanted to return to her own home with her husband, who provided well for her. They used to cook meals together and went to ballroom dancing several times a week until she had moved in with Amelia. Gertrude showed Nurse Robert an article in the local senior center newsletter about an award for ballroom dancing that she and Homer won the week before she moved to Amelia's house. Gertrude confided that Amelia had never "taken to" Homer and frequently tried to discredit their marriage. Gertrude also stated that Homer was an excellent driver and never had any tickets or accidents but that "Amelia would do anything to keep us from going places together." In confidential conversations, Gertrude talked with Nurse Robert about her daughter's controlling behaviors and pleaded for him to help her move back to her own home with her husband. When Nurse Robert talked with Amelia about this possibility, she insisted that her mother's wishes were unreasonable and should not be considered because Gertrude "has dementia and is incapable of knowing what she wants or what is good for her. Besides, Homer is a clever man and he puts on a good front but the only thing he cares about is being able to keep living in my mother's house."

What Nurse Robert Thinks

Although it would be easy to go along with Amelia's viewpoint that Homer cannot provide the care that Gertrude needs, I have serious concerns about this situation. I met Homer several times when he came to church because this was his only opportunity to see Gertrude and they seemed very happy together. She was very affectionate

(continued)

CASE 8.3 When a Family Member Exerts Undue Control Over Plans for an Older Adult *(continued)*

toward him and he was very caring toward her. They looked like a genuinely contented husband and wife. When Homer's daughter was with them, I took the opportunity to ask her privately about the situation. She confirmed my suspicions that Amelia has an agenda that is not in Gertrude's best interests. She also stated that her father is an excellent driver and "he cooks and cleans better than most women do." Homer's daughter has advised him to seek legal help for the situation, but he has not yet followed through on that advice.

What Nurse Robert Does

Nurse Robert reports the situation to adult protective services for investigation. He does not talk with Gertrude or anyone else about the report, but continues to meet with her. Whenever he meets with Gertrude, he documents her statements and his observations. He also documents statements made by Amelia, Homer, and Homer's daughter, recognizing that his assessments will be relevant when legal proceedings occur.

Resolution of Ethical Dilemma

When Nurse Robert used his nursing skills to gather information and "put the puzzle pieces together," he strongly suspected that Gertrude's situation had elements of elder abuse. He appropriately reported the case for investigation and continued as a faith community nurse in an ongoing support role. Despite Nurse Robert's reluctance to get involved with family matters—especially when legal actions may be involved—he acted on his ethical responsibility to advocate for Gertrude's rights.

RESOURCES NURSES CAN USE TO ADDRESS ETHICAL CONCERNS

Health care agencies and institutions have policies and procedures for addressing ethical issues, but elder abuse situations are not always within the scope of these formal resources. In addition, because many of the ethical issues related to elder abuse are subtle and difficult to recognize, they are often overlooked—or simply ignored—in clinical settings. Resolving ethical issues related to elder abuse often calls for creativity on the part of nurses to recommend or suggest referrals for resources that might be effective in addressing these concerns. Adult protective services organizations usually are willing to advise about questionable situations, even without a formal referral for investigation. Similarly, long-term ombudsman programs are usually willing to provide consultation without investigation when ethical concerns are raised about care in long-term care facilities. Nurses can call either of these organizations anonymously and obtain guidance about directions that should be taken when they have questions about specific situations.

When an older adult is receiving care in a hospital setting, specialized geriatric resources can be helpful in addressing ethical issues related to elder abuse. Many hospitals have specialized units or programs for addressing older adults with complex needs using a multidisciplinary approach. Since 1992, the Nurses Improving Care for Healthsystem Elders (NICHE) program has supported the development of geriatric nursing skills for nurses in hospital and other health care settings. In 2016, more than 600 hospitals nationwide were active in the NICHE program, providing education and consultation services by geriatric resource nurses and other geriatric professionals. In addition, social workers are available in all health care settings and they are skilled in identifying resources and making referrals for appropriate services.

When ethical issues emerge during discharge planning—which is often the case—health care professionals are pressured to support the plan that is most readily implemented. When plans involve a discharge to a home or semi-independent setting (e.g., board and care home, or assisted living facility), community-based services can be called upon for follow-up. Nurses do not always make referrals for these services, but they have many opportunities to provide information about these programs to older adults and their families. This is particularly important when risks to elder abuse are detected, and the situation does not meet criteria for reporting to adult protective services.

BECOMING COMFORTABLE WITH ETHICAL ISSUES RELATED TO ELDER ABUSE

By their very nature, ethical issues related to elder abuse are associated with feelings of anxiety and discomfort for all people involved, both professionally and personally. Some situations are "heart breakers" when the circumstances become known and questions are raised about how the disastrous consequences could have been prevented. Even when elder abuse situations do not directly involve ethical issues, health care professionals may be uncomfortable when they need to work with family members or caregivers who have perpetrated the abuse or neglect. This is particularly challenging when health care professionals have questions about the moral character of family members or caregivers who perpetrated the abuse but will continue to be involved.

Professionals also experience feelings of frustration—and even hopelessness—when they are unable to implement a plan that includes any significant and effective interventions. This is particularly frustrating when interventions to resolve some issues are available but the older adult or other people involved with the situation refuse to accept any solutions. Another source of discomfort in elder abuse situations is the difficulty of avoiding "taking sides" with one of the parties involved. Practitioners may overidentify with either the older adult or the perpetrator–caregivers and have difficulty seeing the whole picture. In all situations, professionals have an ethical responsibility to advocate for both the rights of and the provision of appropriate care for the older adult.

When nurses address elder abuse situations, it is important to acknowledge their full range of personal reactions, which can include anger toward family members who are part of the problem. It also is important to recognize personal biases and cultural differences that can influence the practitioner's responses to and feelings about a situation of elder abuse or neglect. An important next step is to use appropriate methods of addressing their feelings about the situation. As with other challenging clinical situations, nurses can share their feelings with colleagues or with other professionals involved with the situation. Another strategy for dealing with one's personal responses to elder abuse is to frequently remind oneself of the inherent right of adults to make decisions about their care. In conjunction with this right, health care professionals are responsible for providing information about a range of choices so patients can make informed decisions. Nurses are in key positions to help develop care plans, including discharge plans, that address risks and respect autonomy, as discussed in Part III.

KEY POINTS: WHAT NURSES NEED TO KNOW AND CAN DO

■ Questions about an older adult's decision making underlie the core ethical issues in many elder abuse situations.

■ *Consent*, *decision-making capacity*, and *undue influence* are legal terms associated with elder abuse (Box 8.1).

■ Clinical assessment of decision-making capacity is a multifaceted process involving considerations such as the person's health, mental status, values, usual lifestyle, cultural influences, and past and current interpersonal relationships.

■ Conclusions about decision-making capacity should not be based solely on age or diagnosis.

■ Although decision-making capacity is determined in clinical settings in relation to specific circumstances, competency is a legal term that is decided through court proceedings and refers to one's overall abilities to fulfill one's roles and handle one's affairs.

■ Adult protective services ethical guidelines emphasize the importance of balancing the duty to protect the safety of the vulnerable adult with the adult's right to self-determination (Box 8.2).

■ Case examples illustrate how nurses address ethical dilemmas in the following types of situations: (a) when the wishes of an older adult conflict with the plans of family caregivers, (b) when there is a conflict between self-determination and safety of an older adult, and (c) when a family member exerts undue control over plans for an older adult.

■ It is important to be familiar with resources for addressing ethical dilemmas associated with elder abuse.

■ Nurses can use information in this chapter to identify self-care strategies for addressing personal anxiety or discomfort that occurs when they care for older adults who are abused.

REFERENCES

American Bar Association. (2014). *Legal issues related to elder abuse: A pocket guide for law enforcement.* Retrieved from www.ambar.org/ElderAbuse Guides.

Anetzberger, G. J. (1982). *Principles of practice in adult protective services.* Presentation at National Elder Abuse Conference, Milwaukee, WI.

National Association of Adult Protective Services (NAPSA). (2004). *Ethical principles and best practices guidelines.* Retrieved from www.napsa-now .org

III

BEYOND KNOWING ABOUT ELDER ABUSE: WHAT NURSES CAN DO TO ADDRESS IT

UNIQUE ASPECTS OF NURSING ASSESSMENT RELATED TO ELDER ABUSE

Elder abuse situations are similar to chronic health conditions in the following respects: (a) Risk factors can usually be identified, (b) the condition develops gradually and initially it may be "asymptomatic" or unobservable to others, and (c) the situation often entails intermittent exacerbations that require medical attention. In other respects, elder abuse situations differ significantly and require nurses to apply assessment skills in unique ways, as in the following aspects:

- Physical findings can often be attributed to other causes with only the most blatant manifestations being unique to elder abuse.
- Assessment of safety has unique characteristics, including identification of immediate or even life-threatening risks, particularly for older adults who live in community settings.
- Situations of elder abuse often involve some element of resistance from the older person and/or caregiver(s).
- Nurses and other health care professionals are responsible for determining whether the situation warrants a report.
- Assessments by nurses and other health care professionals may be essential for determining whether legal interventions are appropriate or necessary for protection of the older adult.

An additional unique aspect in home and community settings is that nurses may be viewed as a threat rather than as a help, and an initial challenge may involve gaining access and obtaining adequate and accurate information. Also, risks to the nurse's personal safety must be assessed, especially when home visits involve contact with a known or suspected perpetrator.

Elder abuse situations challenge nurses to rely on good assessment skills and all levels of nursing knowledge, including intuitive knowing. The purpose of this chapter is to help nurses use assessment skills to identify older adults who are at risk for elder abuse, as well as those who are in abusive situations. Some risks can be addressed through usual nursing interventions, as discussed in Chapter 10, whereas resolution of actual elder abuse situations often requires the involvement of specialized multidisciplinary resources, as discussed in Chapter 11.

In brief, unique aspects related to detection of elder abuse are as follows: (a) putting the pieces together and (b) raising questions about assessment findings that may be indicators of an abusive situation. The following dimensions of nursing assessment in the context of elder abuse are discussed in this chapter: physical assessment, safety and functioning, psychosocial assessment, and assessment of family caregivers and support resources. The intent is to apply usual assessment skills to nursing assessment of older adults in abusive or potentially abusive situations. Nurses can use the information in Box 9.1 as an overall guide to aspects of nursing assessment that are unique to elder abuse.

PHYSICAL ASSESSMENT

Key indicators of neglect, self-neglect, physical abuse, and sexual abuse can be identified through routine physical assessments. For example, the Centers for Medicare & Medicaid have mandated nursing assessment of skin changes for detection of pressure ulcers; this information can be useful for identifying indicators of neglect or self-neglect. At the same time, skin assessment provides essential information about bruises, which can be a major indicator of physical abuse by trusted others. Another assessment aspect within the scope of nursing is identification of indicators of dehydration, malnutrition, and untreated or poorly managed medical conditions. Although these conditions develop for many reasons, they are also strongly associated with many types of elder abuse. A guiding principle related to physical signs is that health care providers who discover physical injuries during the course of an examination should be mindful of elder abuse as

BOX 9.1 Guide to Nursing Assessment Related to Elder Abuse

Provide an environment conducive to assessment
- Assure privacy for one-on-one assessment of the older adult
- Assure as much comfort for the older adult as possible
- Use communication skills to elicit information (discussed in Chapter 7)
- Consider cultural dimensions of elder abuse (discussed in Chapter 5)

Identify indicators
- Although no diagnostic test or physical sign is specific for elder abuse, good assessment skills uncover clues to elder abuse
- Assess each potential indicator within the broader context of the older adult's health, functioning, and overall situation
- Potential indicators of elder abuse that are identified during usual nursing assessments include bruises, fractures, malnutrition, dehydration, pressure ulcers, and evidence related to activities of daily living
- Assessment of safety is essential for identifying the immediacy and type of interventions
- Because elder abuse is often cumulative and progressive, it is important to identify risks before a situation reaches the level of reporting as a suspected case

Document pertinent findings
- Document all findings that can be signs of or risks for elder abuse
- Use evidence-based information to support conclusions that bruises are likely to be inflicted by others rather than accidental (e.g., figure, inside front cover)
- Document skin abnormalities on figures showing both the front and back of the body
- Document discrepancies between different sources, or between explanatory statements and objective evidence
- Document caregiver behaviors that are generally regarded as "red flags" for abusive situations (e.g., caregiver refuses to allow privacy, lack of concern about significant findings)
- Document changes in behavior of the older adult when the caregiver is or is not present (e.g., unwillingness to talk when the caregiver is present, signs of relief when caregiver is not present)
- Review patient records for indicators that were identified during previous encounters and consider these in relation to current assessment information
- Document reports to or activities of adult protective services

a cause. Alternatively, providers who suspect any type of elder abuse should look for signs (Gibbs, 2014).

Any of the following conditions can be indicators of abuse, neglect, or self-neglect: leg ulcers; pressure ulcers; dependent edema; poor wound healing; burns from stoves, cigarettes, or hot water; and bruises, swelling, or injuries from falls, especially repeated falls. More than one of these indicators at the same time, or over a period of time, should raise high levels of suspicion about abuse or neglect. To detect physical abuse, look for evidence of injury caused by others, such as marks from cuts, bites, burns, or punctures, or bruises or injuries, as discussed in the next section.

Bruises and Injuries

Assessment of bruises and injuries is particularly relevant to elder abuse because it is imperative to identify whether the cause was accidental (i.e., unintentional), inflicted by others (i.e., intentional), or self-inflicted (least commonly). Look for bruises that reflect the shape of objects, such as belts or hairbrushes, and patterns of bruises, for example, similar bruises on both upper arms that would result from being grabbed or shaken harshly. If evidence of fall-related injuries is present, consider the possibility that the person was shoved or pushed. Also consider whether the pattern of injuries matches the explanation given by the older adult or caregivers, as in the following examples: (a) bruises or fractures in people who are not ambulatory, (b) a foreword fall in people with Parkinson's disease, who tend to fall backward. Also consider whether falls may be caused by balance and mobility problems due to overmedication by a caregiver (Gibbs, 2014).

Evidence-based information is emerging to help health care professionals identify bruises and injuries that are red flags for abusive situations. For example, a landmark study published by Mosqueda, Burnright, and Liao (2005) identified the most common places for accidental bruises in older adults as extremities (89%) and the dorsal aspect of the arms (76%). A follow-up study of bruising in older adults who were identified as victims of elder abuse resulted in the following characteristics:

■ Bruises were large (e.g., at least one bruise 5 cm [2 in.] in diameter or larger)

■ Bruises could be anywhere, but most often were on the face, arms, or back

- Ninety percent of older adults with bruises that were inflicted by others could tell you how they got their bruises, and this included many older adults with memory problems and dementia. (Wiglesworth et al., 2009).

The figure on inside front cover can serve as an assessment guide to patterns of bruises as reported by abused elders. The authors of this study emphasize the importance of asking older adults about bruises, gently and in private.

A recent study of intentionally caused injuries in older adults presenting to emergency departments found that injuries occurring to the head, neck, or upper trunk and those involving contusions, abrasions, lacerations, or puncture were likely the result of an intentional injury. Moreover, this study found that intentionally injured older adults were much more likely to be struck by or against an object and were less likely to be hospitalized compared with those who were unintentionally injured (Yonashiro-Cho, Gassoumis, & Wilber, 2015).

Pressure Ulcers and Other Skin Indicators

Although pressure ulcers can develop even with good care, they can also be a key indicator of neglect. Important considerations with regard to pressure ulcers are as follows: (a) whether medical care is being provided and treatment has been initiated, (b) whether the treatment is effective, (c) whether caregivers understand how to manage pressure ulcers, and (d) whether caregivers implement interventions to prevent pressure ulcers when the older adult has risk factors (e.g., poor nutrition, limited mobility, exposure of skin to moisture). Skin should also be assessed for indicators of poor hygiene or infections. Body areas that are most commonly neglected are the feet, groin and genital area, and any intertriginous areas (e.g., breast or abdominal folds).

Nutrition and Hydration

Assessment of nutrition and hydration status is important in determining not only the existence of physical neglect but also the seriousness and urgency of the situation. In home and community-based settings, when nurses identify signs of malnutrition or dehydration in older adults, their next step is to determine whether the hydration or nutritional status can be improved sufficiently without removing the person from the setting. For example, simple measures such as provision of home-delivered meals or assistance with grocery shopping and food preparation may alleviate one aspect of situations of self-neglect. Similarly, when older adults are admitted to acute care facilities with either of these diagnoses, it is important to address underlying causes during discharge planning.

Medical Conditions

Older adults who are frail or have medical conditions are likely to develop hypothermia and hyperthermia when exposed to environmental temperatures that are even slightly too cold or too hot. In situations of neglect, caregivers may be responsible for not maintaining comfortable temperatures in living areas. For example, caregivers may not want to spend money for providing adequate heating or cooling or for repairing or replacing equipment that is not functional. In self-neglect situations, older adults may lack the cognitive capacity to sense that temperatures are not appropriate or to operate thermostats properly.

Infections can also be a sign of elder abuse, as in the following examples:

- Untreated and infected skin conditions, including wounds, leg ulcers, and pressure ulcers, due to neglect or self-neglect
- Recurrent urinary tract infections, due to sexual abuse or poorly managed incontinence
- Aspiration pneumonia, due to inappropriate feeding methods used by caregivers
- Sexually transmitted infections, due to sexual abuse

As with all aspects of assessment of older adults in abusive situations, these conditions need to be considered within the broader context.

ASSESSMENT OF SAFETY AND FUNCTIONING

Assessment of safety in the context of elder abuse is both essential and wide ranging. It is essential because the choice of legal interventions is influenced in part by the degree of risk and the decision-making capacity of the older adult, as discussed in Chapter 8. It is wide ranging because safety issues are related not only to protection from abuse or neglect perpetrated by others, but also to self-neglect for older adults who live alone. It is also wide ranging because consequences may be relatively harmless or they may cause irreparable damage or even death if risks are not identified and addressed.

Elder abuse situations often require an immediate determination of the degree to which the conditions are life-threatening or pose significant risks to health. In emergency departments, nursing assessments of the broader situations and risks to safety may provide essential information that influences plans for admission or discharge. In domestic elder abuse situations, it is imperative to assess the degree to which the family members or caregivers present a threat to the life of the dependent older person.

In home care settings, nurses are often the first-line health care professionals called upon to assess the situation. For example, when situations are first discovered, questions may arise about removing the person from the environment. Many times, however, the person may not want to leave, or there may be no better setting in which the person can receive care immediately. In these situations, nurses may be asked to assess the urgency and seriousness of the situation and to provide an opinion about whether legal interventions should be considered. In addition, the nurse often is the person who can either convince the older adult to accept help or convince the caregivers and social workers that the present situation is tolerable. For instance, when nurses determine that the conditions are not life-threatening, they can reassure the older adult that they are trying to improve the situation so the older adult remains as safe and independent as possible.

Safety concerns in some situations address risks not only to the older adult but also to other people and properties due to unsafe behaviors of the older adult, for example, with unsafe smoking or driving. Protection of one's assets is a safety concern that is addressed in Chapter 15. Nurses can use Box 9.2 as a guide to assessment of safety concerns pertinent to elder abuse situations.

Assessment of Medication Management

Nurses routinely assess a patient's ability to manage medical conditions, and in some situations of elder abuse this is an aspect of safety. For example, consequences can be quite serious when a person with diabetes or heart failure does not take medications correctly and lives alone. When a medication regimen is complex, it is important to determine if it can be simplified to improve adherence and support the person's ability to remain in an independent setting. For example, in institutional settings medications might be administered four or more

BOX 9.2 Guide to Assessment of Safety Related to Elder Abuse

Concerns related to personal safety

- History of physical abuse on the part of the caregiver or family member, especially when the older adult is unable to escape or otherwise be protected
- Environmental conditions in the living environment or neighborhood associated with undue risk for disease, physical harm, hypothermia, hyperthermia, or becoming a victim of crime
- Repeated episodes of getting lost or wandering in unsafe neighborhoods or in very cold weather without proper clothing
- History of frequent falls, especially if explanations do not match patterns of injuries or if the person lives alone and cannot call for help

Concerns related to health

- Untreated or poorly managed medical conditions
- Untreated wounds or infections
- Serious and untreated injuries
- Inability to meet basic needs (e.g., nutrition, hydration, personal hygiene, urinary and bowel elimination)
- Inappropriate use of drugs or alcohol, either self- or caregiver-induced
- Inability to recognize personal emergency situations and call for help, particularly in combination with high-risk conditions, such as frequent falls, physically abusive caregivers, and unstable medical conditions
- Suicide potential, especially in self-neglected elders who are also depressed and expressing feelings of hopelessness
- Access to toxic substances or dangerous tools or cutlery in the household without the ability to recognize the dangers

Concerns involving risks to self and others due to unsafe behaviors of the older adult

- Unsafe driving of vehicles
- Unsafe use of appliances (e.g., gas stoves)
- Unsafe smoking (e.g., falling asleep with lighted cigarette)
- Access to weapons without the ability to make safe and appropriate decisions about their use

different times during a 24-hour period. However, even though this might be ideal, people in home settings may not be able to follow this regimen, particularly if the older adult lives alone and requires assistance with medications.

Another assessment consideration is that elder abuse may involve caregivers withholding therapeutic medications or interfering with medical care. For example, caregivers may decide not to purchase prescriptions or provide nursing care, medical equipment, or comfort items because they do not want to spend the money, even though this care is recommended and even prescribed. If the older adult has not freely chosen to forego treatments, medications, or assistance, then this may constitute neglect. If the caregiver is likely to inherit the money that is being saved, this may represent financial exploitation as well.

Relationship Between Functional Abilities and Risks to Safety

In elder abuse situations, nursing assessment focuses on the relationship between functional abilities and risks to safety, as in the following examples:

- In certain medical conditions, one's ability to follow medical regimens can have serious outcomes, for example, when a person with diabetes or heart failure does not take medications correctly.
- Bowel and bladder incontinence in people who are confined to bed or a chair can increase the risk for pressure ulcers.
- People with mobility limitations, balance problems, or serious visual impairments can be at increased risk for falls.

Similarly, nurses need to consider whether frailty creates risks for safety in elder abuse situations. For example, in self-neglect situations, an older adult who is physically healthy and fully ambulatory would not have the same degree of risk for fall-related injuries as one who weighs only 78 lbs. and ambulates unsteadily with a walker. Similarly, if the 75-year-old wife of an alcoholic man can easily escape to safety when he becomes violent, and she chooses to remain in the situation, she would not necessarily be considered a protective case. In contrast, if the woman's decision-making capacity is questionable, and she is frail, cognitively impaired, or unable to move quickly, and is the target of violence when her husband is inebriated, the situation could be defined as elder abuse.

Relationship Between Assessment of Safety and Acceptance of Interventions

When risks to safety are identified in elder abuse situations, the next step is to implement interventions, as discussed in Chapter 10. A major assessment consideration in these situations is determining the extent to which the older adult is willing to accept interventions. If the older adult refuses to accept recommendations, the next step is to assess the person's decision-making capacity, which can be an ongoing process, as illustrated in Figure 9.1.

PSYCHOSOCIAL ASSESSMENT

Decision-making capacity, which is an essential component of psychosocial assessment, is often the core issue when older adults express the desire to continue living in a situation that involves risks, as discussed in Chapter 8. This chapter discusses the following aspects of psychosocial assessment related to elder abuse: dementia, depression, the right to refuse services, the influence of drugs or alcohol, and psychological consequences of being in an abusive situation. Nursing interventions to address these issues are discussed in Chapter 10.

Dementia, Depression, and the Right to Refuse Services

As discussed in Parts I and II of this book, dementia is strongly associated with an increased risk for elder abuse in many ways. A unique aspect of dementia in relation to elder abuse is that families or caregivers may inaccurately report that a person has dementia or they may intentionally provide false information about an older adult's abilities as a way of gaining control over assets and dominating decisions about care. Thus, it is imperative to objectively assess the effects of dementia on safety, functioning, and risk for abuse and to raise questions about observations that are not consistent with information provided by the family. Depression is also associated with elder abuse in many ways and should be assessed as a potentially treatable condition. Studies suggest depression is related to elder abuse in a bidirectional way: being a victim of abuse or neglect may be a stressor leading to depression, and being depressed may increase the older adult's vulnerability to abuse and neglect as well as to decreased likelihood of reporting abuse (Cooper & Livingston, 2014). Nurses can use Box 9.3 as a guide to psychosocial assessment related to older adults in abusive situations.

FIGURE 9.1   Relationship between assessment of safety and acceptance of interventions.

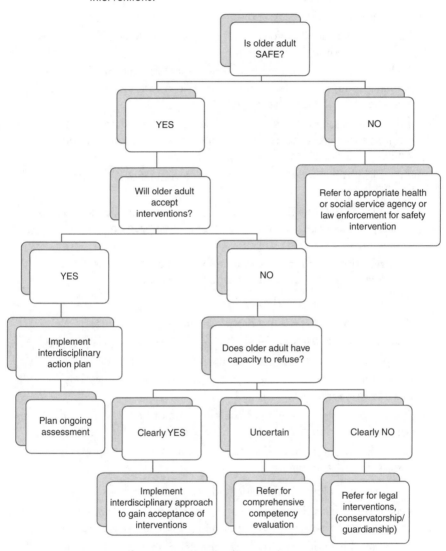

Considerations Related to the Influence of Drugs or Alcohol

The possibility of substance abuse by the older adult should also be considered in all situations of suspected abuse or self-neglect, especially if the older adult is depressed, grieving, socially isolated, or has a history of substance abuse. Nurses also assess effects of inappropriate use or administration of psychoactive medications, either by the

BOX 9.3 Guide to Psychosocial Assessment Related to Elder Abuse

Considerations related to dementia
- Does the older adult have a diagnosis of dementia?
- Does the older adult have signs or symptoms of dementia and, if so, has any evaluation been done?
- Do family members express concerns about the older adult having dementia and, if so, are the concerns valid or are they associated with ulterior motives of the family?
- If the older adult has a diagnosis of dementia, do others use this diagnosis to impose decisions or control assets that are not consistent with the older adult's wishes?
- If the older adult has dementia, to what extent does it increase the risk for abuse?
- If the older adult has dementia, to what extent does it affect decision making or any aspect of safety, including management of medical conditions and protection of assets?
- How do caregivers manage dementia-associated behaviors (e.g., dependency, aggression, psychiatric manifestations)?

Considerations related to depression
- Does the older adult have a diagnosis or history of depression?
- Does the older adult have signs or symptoms of depression (e.g., flat or sad affect, excessive crying, loss of appetite, unintentional weight loss)?
- If the older adult has signs or symptoms of depression, has any evaluation been done?
- Does depression, or feelings of helplessness or hopelessness, interfere with the older adult obtaining or accepting outside services?
- Is the older adult at risk for suicide, and, if so, have precautions or interventions been initiated?

Considerations related to the older adult's right to refuse services
- If the older adult's decision-making capacity is questionable, has a comprehensive evaluation been done by qualified professionals?
- Does the older adult acknowledge the need for support resources?
- Does the older adult express a willingness to use recommended services?
- Does the older adult understand the consequences of not accepting services?
- What are the barriers to the older adult accepting services (see Box 9.4)?

older adult or imposed by caregivers. Sometimes caregivers who abuse drugs or alcohol will give these substances to the people for whom they care, especially if the dependent person is not able or willing to refuse. Another circumstance associated with elder abuse is the use of excessive amounts of psychoactive medications solely for the caregiver's benefit to control behaviors of the older adult. Nurses are likely to observe any of the following indicators of overmedication in an elder: confusion, slurred speech, excessive sleeping, problems with balance or mobility, or neurological adverse effects.

Considerations Related to Emotional Consequences of Elder Abuse

Nurses are in key positions to assess emotional consequences of elder abuse, which are often overlooked even when they are serious. It is also important to recognize that people with dementia can remember—and experience emotional consequences of—events such as abuse that have strong emotional content (Wiglesworth & Mosqueda, 2009). Nurses can use communication techniques discussed in Chapter 7 to encourage older adults to express their feelings about their situations.

ASSESSMENT OF CAREGIVERS AND SUPPORT RESOURCES

The term *caregivers* is used to describe all the people, including family members, kinship network, friends, paid caregivers, and trusted others, upon whom the older adult relies for assistance and emotional support. The term *support resources* describes people and services who could provide assistance and emotional support. In self-neglect situations, support resources are absent or minimal, for reasons such as lack of available services or unacceptability on the part of the older adult. In domestic elder abuse situations, major conflicts may exist among those who are involved in the care of a dependent older adult and those who are willing to provide support but are excluded for a variety of reasons. In addition, some or all of the caregivers may directly cause the abusive situation or may actively or passively contribute to it. When the people who perpetrate the abuse are also the support resources, nurses assess the potential for working with them to prevent further abuse. It is not always easy to work with abusive caregivers, but it may be even more difficult to eliminate their influence over an older adult. For example, an alcoholic son may live with his mother who has early-stage dementia and provide emotional support and minimal assistance with care but also financially exploit her and neglect her safety needs.

In addition, nursing assessment focuses on barriers to using support resources that are potential sources of assistance or support but are not currently being used. Box 9.4 delineates guidelines for nursing assessment of social supports in relation to elder abuse situations.

BOX 9.4 Guide to Nursing Assessment of Social Supports

Considerations related to the older adult's perceptions of, and attitudes and knowledge about, support resources

- What does the older adult know about services that are available?
- What financial assets are available for support resources and is the older adult willing to use them?
- Does the older adult feel that family is the only acceptable source of care?
- Does the older adult mistrust service providers?
- Has the older adult had bad experiences with service providers or heard about bad experiences of others?
- Do language or cultural barriers interfere with the use of services?
- Do concerns about accessibility or transportation present barriers to obtaining health care or using community-based services?
- Does the older adult fear that the home situation will be judged as socially unacceptable?

Considerations related to support resources already involved

- What support resources are currently involved (e.g., family, friends, kinship network, local aging services, religion-based organization)?
- Are any of the caregivers also the perpetrators of abuse?
- Are any of the caregivers involved primarily for personal gain (e.g., greed, financial exploitation)?
- Do the people who are involved with caregiving have conflicts about their involvement (e.g., sense of obligation that causes excessive stress or risks to own health)?
- What are the strengths of the caregivers (e.g., availability, family loyalty and support, positive relationships)?
- What are the weaknesses of the caregivers (e.g., greed, mental health problems, lack of caregiving skills)?
- Are the caregivers willing to change the situation (e.g., accept outside resources, learn appropriate caregiving skills)?

Assessment of Family Caregivers in Relation to Needs of the Older Adult

Nurses routinely assess family caregivers, with a focus on teaching them how to manage care to the extent necessary for, and appropriate to, the situation. In some elder abuse situations, an added dimension is assessing caregivers who also may be perpetrating abuse or increasing the risk for abuse. The case example in Chapter 14 illustrates ways in which nurses work as an integral part of an interdisciplinary team to identify and address risks in caregivers to prevent elder abuse. This chapter focuses on ways in which nurses assess caregivers and family members who are actual or potential perpetrators of abuse, and Chapter 10 describes nursing interventions associated with the identified needs. An important assessment aspect is identifying strengths of the overall situation that can be built upon with interventions. This is especially important when the situation involves a caregiver who perpetrates abuse, either intentionally or unintentionally.

In clinical settings, nurses have many opportunities to interact with family caregivers when they accompany older adults to appointments or visit in institutional settings. Asking open-ended questions about the needs of the caregivers can lead to information that can be used to develop interventions. This may be particularly effective when caregivers unintentionally perpetrate abusive situations or create risks for abuse because of their lack of skills and information or their own emotional needs. Nurses can use Box 9.5 as a guide to assessment of family caregivers in relation to elder abuse situations.

BOX 9.5 Guide to Nursing Assessment of Family Caregivers

Considerations related to mental health issues of caregivers

- Is there evidence of drug or alcohol abuse in the caregiver?
- Has the caregiver been diagnosed with dementia or a mental illness (e.g., depression, schizophrenia, or anxiety disorder)?

Considerations related to stress and coping of caregivers

- Does the caregiver indicate that he or she is experiencing major stressors in his or her life, in addition to the stresses related to caregiving?
- Does the caregiver indicate that he or she feels undue stress from multiple demands and responsibilities?

(continued)

BOX 9.5 Guide to Nursing Assessment of Family Caregivers *(continued)*

Considerations related to strengths and weaknesses of caregivers

- Are caregivers receptive to interventions related to improving caregiving skills?
- What sources of support—for both the caregiver and the older adult—are acceptable to the caregiver?
- What are the barriers to the caregiver's use of support resources?

Questions to ask caregivers

- "What effects does this situation have on . . . your health . . . your immediate family? . . . your work life? . . . your quality of life? . . . your marriage?"
- "How do you cope with stress?"
- "How is your health?"
- "Are you overlooking your own needs because of this situation?"

KEY POINTS: WHAT NURSES NEED TO KNOW AND CAN DO

- Bruises, pressure ulcers, nutrition and hydration status, and medical conditions need to be assessed in the context of the broader situation to determine whether these conditions are associated with elder abuse.

- Nurses assess safety and functioning in relation to risks for elder abuse and in relation to acceptance of intervention.

- Dementia, depression, and decision-making abilities are assessed in relation to risks and interventions for older adults in abusive situations.

- Psychosocial assessment related to elder abuse includes considerations about the emotional consequences and the possible influence of drugs and alcohol.

- Assessment of caregivers and social supports in elder abuse situations is imperative for identifying contributing conditions that can be addressed through interventions.

- It is important to observe communication between older adults and spouses, partners, friends, and family members to identify interpersonal issues that can be addressed.

- Nurses need to arrange for private assessment of the older adult and consider the need for private conversations with families or caregivers.

- It is imperative to document concerns, observations, assessment findings, and pertinent statements of the older adult and others.

REFERENCES

Cooper, C., & Livingston, G. (2014). Mental health/psychiatric issues in elder abuse and neglect. *Clinics in Geriatric Medicine, 30*, 839–850.

Gibbs, L. M. (2014). Understanding the medical markers of elder abuse and neglect: Physical examination findings. *Clinics in Geriatric Medicine, 30*, 687–712.

Mosqueda, L., Burnright, K., & Liao, S. (2005). The life cycle of bruises in older adults. *Journal of the American Geriatrics Society, 53*, 1339–1343.

Wiglesworth, A., Austin, R., Corona, M., Schneider, D., Liao, S., Gibbs, L., & Mosqueda, L. (2009). Bruising as a marker of physical elder abuse. *Journal of the American Geriatrics Society, 57*, 1191–1196.

Wiglesworth, A., & Mosqueda, L. (2009). *People with dementia as witnesses to emotional events*. Final Technical Report to the U.S. Department of Justice. Retrieved from www.ncjrs.gov/pdffiles1/nij/grants/234132.pdf

Yonashiro-Cho, J., Gassoumis, Z., & Wilber, K. (2015, November 19). *Characteristics of intentional injuries among older adults presenting to hospital emergency departments in 2001–2010*. Presentation at Gerontological Society of America Scientific Meeting, Orlando, FL.

UNIQUE ASPECTS OF NURSING INTERVENTIONS RELATED TO ELDER ABUSE

OVERALL APPROACH TO NURSING INTERVENTIONS RELATED TO ELDER ABUSE

In health care settings, interventions for elder abuse focus on the following: (a) addressing risk factors and contributing conditions, (b) managing or reducing consequences, and (c) preventing further abuse. Although complex and multidisciplinary interventions are required in many elder abuse situations, nurses can draw on commonly used nursing interventions to address elder abuse in health care settings. Interventions discussed in this chapter are relevant to nurses who provide care for older adults in any clinical setting, including medical offices, hospitals, emergency departments, hospice and palliative care programs, and homes and community-based settings. In addition, nurses have important roles in suggesting or facilitating referrals for community-based resources to address the broader issues inherent in many elder abuse situations, as described in Chapter 11.

Some aspects of elder abuse are addressed through interventions that are well within the scope of usual nursing practice, such as in the following examples:

- Treating injuries and pressure ulcers
- Managing medical conditions
- Teaching about medication management

- Teaching about interventions for safe and optimal functioning
- Improving knowledge of caregivers related to care

In addition to these usual nursing interventions, interventions for elder abuse situations often require nurses to address contributing circumstances such as dysfunctional family dynamics, limitations of the caregivers, resistance to changing an abusive situation, and other challenges inherent in the situation. Another consideration in many situations is that it may be difficult to respect the autonomy of older adults when their decisions support a situation that is viewed as unhealthy, unsafe, or risky.

Another challenge for nurses is that there are few evidence-based interventions specifically related to care of older adults who are in abusive situations or at risk for elder abuse. This is particularly true for hospital settings, where protocols for addressing elder abuse tend to focus on identification and reporting, rather than on direct interventions (DuMont et al., 2015). A recent review of 62 studies of abuse and neglect of older adults emphasized the need for interventions to be multipronged, individualized, coordinated, interprofessional, emotionally supportive, culturally considerate, patient-centered, acceptable to all involved, and focused on reduction of harm (Hirst et al., 2016). This recommendation may seem idealistic, but, in reality, many nursing interventions are effective for addressing the needs of older adults who are in abusive or potentially abusive situations. Thus, this chapter describes the many ways in which nurses can use nursing skills to address the complexities of elder abuse when caring for older adults in clinical settings.

APPLYING USUAL NURSING INTERVENTIONS TO ELDER ABUSE SITUATIONS

Building Trust

An essential first step for successfully implementing interventions for elder abuse is establishing a trusting relationship between the older adult and a professional service provider. Nurses who provide short-term or intermittent care for an older adult may not have opportunities to address the situation on an ongoing basis, but they can establish a trusting relationship that becomes the "bridge" to service providers who can implement interventions. For example, when older adults are admitted to hospitals, they may be more receptive to accepting support resources and they may appreciate the input of a health care professional who can talk with their family about the use of support resources. Similarly, when older adults receive outpatient care, nurses have intermittent but ongoing opportunities to build on a trusting relationship that opens the door to communication about abusive situations.

Nurses are in key positions to talk with older adults and family caregivers about the use of support resources as interventions for a stressful or abusive situation. Rather than directly referring to abuse, nurses can phrase the conversation in the context of preventing and addressing health issues for both the older adults and family caregivers. Older adults and caregivers may respond to this nonthreatening approach, especially if the health of the older adult has been jeopardized by the caregiving situation or the lack of care or social supports.

Establishing Realistic Goals

Identifying realistic goals for nursing care is an early and ongoing challenge when caring for older adults in abusive situations because of the complexity of the situation and the resistance to services commonly encountered by health care professionals. As discussed in Chapter 8, ethical dilemmas are associated with situations involving conflicts between the right of the older adult to choose risks, relationships, and living conditions, and the recommendations of health care professionals related to safety and health care. Although nurses should not assume that older adults and caregivers will resist the use of services or a move to another setting, they need to be prepared to address resistance on both the part of the older adult and the caregivers, who also may be the perpetrators. In these situations, the limited goal may be to respect the person's autonomy and prevent risk to the extent that is realistic. Even with this limited goal, however, professionals who are addressing the situation generally try to convince the older adult or family caregivers to voluntarily address the risks. Ultimately, however, all those involved, including health care professionals and adult protective service workers, may need to accept a very limited goal of respecting autonomy.

Addressing Resistance

An approach that has been used to address resistance in elder abuse situations is based on the Stages of Change model developed by Prochaska and DiClemente (1982), which is widely applied to promote healthier behaviors. The Eliciting Change in At-Risk Elders (ECARE) model applies behavior-change principles to chronic and change-resistant elder abuse situations by matching interventions to stages of change as follows:

- Precontemplation stage (i.e., no desire): encourage older adults to discuss issues and acknowledge harmful effects they experience.

- Contemplation stage (ambivalence): discuss costs and benefits of making change, and develop a plan for safety, if applicable.

- Preparation stage: educate older adults about available resources and address barriers to action.

- Action stage: help older adults connect with support resources or make constructive changes, while helping them overcome obstacles and frustrations.

- Maintenance state: help older adults recognize gains and develop plans for preventing recurrence (Mariam, McClure, Robinson, & Yang, 2015).

A study of older adults at risk for elder abuse found that this approach effectively reduced abuse-related risk factors, empowering the participants to move toward enhanced safety and autonomy (Mariam et al., 2015). An important implication is that nursing interventions may help older adults move to the next stage of change, even if they do not immediately move to the action or maintenance stage. Thus, any interventions directed toward resolution or prevention of elder abuse may have subtle and long-term benefits that nurses may not recognize during the course of providing short-term care.

Addressing Behavioral and Mental Health Issues

Much evidence points toward high rates of depression, anxiety disorders, alcohol abuse, psychological distress, poor mental health, and posttraumatic stress disorders in older adults who are or have been in abusive situations (Cooper & Livingston, 2014; Sirey et al., 2015). Mental health professionals can address these consequences by providing counseling about handling abusive situations and managing the psychological effects of abuse. Nurses have key roles in talking with older adults about mental health issues and discussing pertinent resources.

Dementia is strongly associated with an increased risk for elder abuse, particularly when dementia-associated behaviors are present. Many health care settings have professionals available for consultation about management of dementia-associated behaviors and nurses can initiate referrals for these resources (discussed in the section "Using

Resources Within Health Care Settings"). A Model Intervention for Elder Abuse and Dementia identified educational and support services for caregivers of people with dementia as an effective intervention for addressing elder abuse (Anetzberger et al., 2000). Nurses can encourage caregivers to explore this type of resource by contacting the local Alzheimer's Association and aging network programs. Box 10.1 delineates nursing interventions to address behavioral and mental health issues related to elder abuse.

Teaching About Self-Protection

Domestic elder abuse situations may involve a significant risk for physical abuse, including sexual abuse, by a spouse, family member, caregiver, or any trusted other. When an older adult chooses to remain in an abusive relationship, health care professionals need to respect this choice as long as the person's decision-making capacity has been evaluated and the person has not been deemed incompetent. Despite the limited goals inherent in these situations, nurses can discuss self-protection interventions, such as developing an escape plan, before a crisis occurs. Also, nurses can discuss the importance of establishing and maintaining quick access to a one-button emergency alert system (e.g., on a cell phone or portable device). In addition, it is important to teach about community-based resources, such as the ones described in Chapter 11.

USING RESOURCES WITHIN HEALTH CARE SETTINGS

Resources Within Acute Care Settings

When elder abuse is identified in acute care settings, specialized geriatric resources may be available to provide direct care or consultation to the nursing staff. In addition, rehabilitation therapists are often overlooked as professional resources for addressing many issues related to elder abuse. Nurses providing care in medical, surgical, or intensive care units can consider requesting a consultation for services that are generally available within health care settings, as delineated in Box 10.2.

Resources in Home and Community-Based Settings

When nurses in home and community-based settings identify elder abuse situations, they may need to be creative in finding other professionals with whom they can work. For example, when working with

BOX 10.1   Nursing Interventions to Address Behavioral and Mental Health Issues Related to Elder Abuse

Nursing interventions to address mental health issues

- Use communication techniques to elicit feelings of the older adult about the abusive situation, including feelings about the perpetrator.
- Validate the feelings of the older adult, while at the same time raising questions about those that have negative effects (e.g., anger, shame, self-blame, helplessness, worthlessness).
- Emphasize that the older adult is not responsible for the actions of others, including family members who perpetrate abuse.
- Explore the effects of the situation on the older adult and help identify ways in which the psychological effects can be addressed.
- Identify unhealthy methods that the older adult may be using to cope with the situation (e.g., alcohol, medications, overeating, social isolation) and discuss the older adult's willingness to address these behaviors.
- Explore ways in which the older adult can apply his or her usual healthy methods of coping to diminish the stress of his or her abusive situation (e.g., support groups, body–mind interventions, spiritually based interventions).
- Explore the role of religion in relation to coping with the abusive situation and support the use of religiously oriented resources as appropriate.
- Discuss the use of mental health professionals or support groups for management of anxiety, depression, substance abuse, posttraumatic stress, or other effects of elder abuse.
- Identify and address barriers to the use of mental health services and community-based programs.

Nursing interventions to address issues related to dementia

- Facilitate referrals for professionals who can address dementia-associated behaviors, including identification of treatable contributing conditions (e.g., depression, medical problems, environmental factors).
- Suggest that older adults and caregivers explore resources provided by the local Alzheimer's Association (contact www.alz.org to find a local contact).
- Suggest the use of community-based services for persons with dementia (respite, adult day care, home care).

BOX 10.2 Services Generally Available in Health Care Settings

Resources for overall assessment of actual or potential elder abuse situations
- Adult and gerontological advanced practice nurses
- Geriatric resource nurses
- Geriatric assessment programs
- Geriatric behavioral health programs

Consultations and evaluations about decision-making capacity
- Geriatric assessment programs
- Geropsychiatrists
- Geropsychologists
- Ethics committees

Rehabilitation therapists for assessment and recommendations related to safety and self-care
- Physical therapists: assessment of and recommendations about functioning and safety, particularly regarding mobility, balance, and prevention of falls
- Occupational therapists: assessment of and recommendations related to safety, self-care, and cognitive abilities
- Speech therapists: assessment of and recommendations related to communication, cognitive abilities, swallowing problems, and feeding and eating techniques to prevent aspiration

Social services
- Assessment of family dynamics and issues related to caregiving
- Assessment and recommendations about long-term care or community-based services
- Assistance with identifying resources for care, including those that are culturally appropriate

older adults who will not or cannot leave the house, nurses need to identify resources for initial and ongoing medical evaluation and care. Primary care providers in many areas of the country are resuming the practice of making home visits. Also, some medical centers or teaching hospitals provide in-home services, including in-home medical evaluations, through their geriatric assessment programs. In addition, with the growing demand for home health services, an increased number of diagnostic tests are performed in the home (e.g., radiography, blood tests, electrocardiography). In many situations, these diagnostic tests are essential for determining whether involuntary care measures are justified. For instance, if the older adult is homebound for any reason, blood tests or radiography done in the home may provide the evidence needed to determine whether a hospitalization is warranted.

Telehealth resources may be available to provide consultations about older adults in home situations. For example, visiting nurse associations, public health nurses, and adult protective service agencies may have access to consultations by using laptop computers or other portable devices. Also, telehealth resources are increasingly being used to monitor home situations and improve the safety of older adults; these may be helpful when addressing actual or potential elder abuse situations. These resources can be particularly helpful when caring for older adults in rural or geographically isolated areas.

Another consideration with regard to some home settings is identifying interventions for the nurse's self-protection. In any situation that places a nurse at risk, it is essential to ensure that appropriate protections and precautions are in place. For example, nurses can arrange their visits in conjunction with protective service workers, or, if warranted, law enforcement officers. Some communities have law enforcement officers who are specially trained to deal with elder abuse situations and are available to accompany service providers. In addition, it is imperative that nurses are vigilant about potential risks and attentive to an escape route. They also need to have access to emergency help, for example, by keeping a cell phone handy and programmed with a one-button emergency call number.

ADDRESSING RISKS TO THE SAFETY OF OTHERS

Domestic elder abuse situations may pose significant risks to the safety of others, such as by causing fires or vehicular accidents. These situations may involve ethical issues and reports to adult protective services if the older adult resists voluntary interventions. Nurses have important roles in suggesting resources for professional assessment of driving and other aspects of functioning. For example, a referral for an occupational therapy evaluation can be an important intervention for addressing overall safety issues, including issues that place others at risk. An approach that may be effective is to discuss the resources

CASE 10.1 Mr. Wilson, Driving Unsafely

Nurse Stella is a faith-based community nurse who works at the First Baptist Circle of Care; she provides counseling and advocacy for concerns related to health. Mr. and Mrs. Wilson, who are members of the congregation, have frequently talked to Nurse Stella about Mr. Wilson's declining health. Mrs. Wilson reports that Mr. Wilson has received five tickets for traffic violations in the last 2 months, but "they were for little things like going through a stop sign or going 30 miles per hour in a 25 miles per hour zone." He has not had any accidents, but the local authorities have contacted his physician and a driving evaluation has been ordered, but neither Mr. nor Mrs. Wilson is in favor of the evaluation. Mr. Wilson says, "They're just out to get me because I'm 87 years old and they have a gripe against me. I know they just want to take away my license and then we'll both be prisoners in our own house." Nurse Stella suspects that Mrs. Wilson expresses support for her husband's viewpoint because she has never driven and they do not want to depend on anyone else for transportation. Nurse Stella says, "The purpose of an evaluation by a driving rehabilitation specialist is to identify ways in which you can improve your driving. It is not their intent to take away your license, but to protect your right to drive as long as you are safe. They also teach you about safe driving and this will help you maintain your independence, which I know is important for you."

as a way of improving functioning and supporting the person's independence. Using this approach, nurses may be able to gain cooperation when older adults view referrals for assessment of safety as a threat to their autonomy, as in the example shown in Case 10.1.

ADDRESSING THE NEEDS OF CAREGIVERS

Situations of neglect may arise from misconceptions or lack of knowledge about providing care for a dependent older adult. Nurses have key roles in identifying abusive or neglectful behaviors that can be addressed by teaching caregivers, as in the examples delineated in Box 10.3. In addition to teaching caregivers, nurses can role model and demonstrate good care while caregivers are present. Nurses can

BOX 10.3 Nursing Interventions to Address Caregiver Issues

Examples of abusive or neglectful actions that can be addressed by nurses

- Caregivers may use adult briefs for managing urinary incontinence without understanding the importance of changing them frequently to prevent skin breakdown.
- Caregivers may not be knowledgeable about alleviating pressure areas to prevent skin breakdown.
- Caregivers may inappropriately restrict fluid intake for the older adult in an effort to reduce urinary incontinence.
- Caregivers may administer excessive amounts of as-needed psychoactive medications because they do not understand the correct dosing schedule or the potential adverse effects.
- Caregivers may have difficulty administering medications correctly because the regimen is too complex.
- Caregivers may use physical restraints inappropriately and unsafely, with the false expectation of reducing falls.

Nursing interventions to address caregiver stress

- Use communication techniques to elicit feelings and expectations about caregiving responsibilities.
- Communicate empathy for the caregiver role and emphasize the importance of self-care.
- Validate the feelings of the caregiver, while at the same time questioning the inappropriate expression of feelings (e.g., physical abuse of the older adult due to anger or impatience).
- Ask caregivers about any positive effects or benefits of caregiving (including financial benefits).
- Identify unhealthy methods that the caregiver may be using to cope with the situation (e.g., alcohol, medications, overeating, social isolation) and discuss his or her willingness to address these behaviors.
- Explore ways in which the caregiver can apply his or her usual healthy methods of coping to diminish the stress of the abusive situation (e.g., support groups, body–mind interventions, spiritually based interventions).
- Discuss the use of professionals and support groups for management of mental health issues such as anxiety, depression, or substance abuse.
- Explore the role of religion in relation to coping with caregiving and support the use of religiously oriented resources as appropriate.
- Identify and address barriers to the use of mental health services.

also include caregivers during direct-care activities and use these as teaching opportunities. Another nursing intervention to improve care in situations of neglect is to initiate referrals for services of other professionals who can address aspects of neglect, such as registered dieticians or rehabilitation therapists. Community-based organizations such as the aging services network or the Alzheimer's Association often provide educational programs for caregivers. Nurses are in unique positions to identify caregiver needs and facilitate referrals for services within institutional settings as well as for follow-up after discharge.

If the caregiver is feeling burdened with caregiving responsibilities, then respite, along with individual or group support and counseling, may be an effective intervention. In mutually abusive situations in which the designated caregiver, often a spouse, is also abused or neglected, the nurse tries to identify any outside sources of support that have not been tapped. For example, in a mutually abusive situation involving a socially isolated married couple, the nurse might identify a relative, friend, or paid caregiver who is willing to provide appropriate assistance. Consider that culturally specific or religion-based resources may be acceptable, when other resources are not. Box 10.3 describes nursing interventions that are appropriate for addressing caregiver issues. In addition, a relatively simple intervention is to express support for efforts of family caregivers, who may feel that their efforts are inadequate or unappreciated.

> I have an older sister and two brothers, and all they can do is call to complain that things aren't getting done right for my mother. They never say "thank you" for what I'm doing. So if I'm doing such a terrible job, maybe I'll just stop doing it. (Gelman, Sokoloff, Graziani, Arias, & Peralta, 2014, p. 673)

CASE 10.2 Nurse Cheryl Addresses Caregiver Needs

Nurse Cheryl is caring for Mrs. Daven, who is 83 years old and has been admitted for pneumonia and has additional diagnoses of hypertension, obesity, and osteoarthritis. Although she had both knees replaced 2 years ago, her mobility is limited due to hip problems. Nurse Cheryl notes that Mrs. Daven is very demanding when her

(continued)

CASE 10.2　Nurse Cheryl Addresses Caregiver Needs *(continued)*

daughter, Ruth, comes to visit and asks for assistance with simple tasks, such as adjusting her bedcovers and changing the channels on the television. When Mrs. Daven's sons visit, she is pleasant and does not ask for help. After visiting her mother, Ruth finds Nurse Cheryl at the nurses' station and asks if they can talk in the conference room. Ruth confides that she is worn out by going to her mother's house 5 days a week and being expected to prepare meals, clean the house, help with personal care, and drive her mother to wherever she wants to go. Ruth says her three brothers and their wives take turns having her mother to their houses for Sunday dinners, but they are not expected to do anything else. Ruth says, "I've come close to hitting my mother a couple times after she yelled at me and told me that I'm the only one of her four children who doesn't have a respectable job and the least I can do is take care of her. If she keeps this up after she gets out of the hospital, I'll probably lose my temper. I feel like such a bad daughter and she just wants more and more out of me." Nurse Cheryl tells Ruth that she will ask the social worker to meet with Mrs. Daven and all the family members for a discharge conference to discuss the many resources for home-based services.

ADDRESSING FAMILY DYNAMICS

An aspect that is more unique to elder abuse is addressing the psychological consequences and interpersonal relationships that are inherent in many of these situations. Domestic elder abuse situations typically involve a broken-trust relationship that affects the older adult in many ways. Even if the perpetrator is or was a stranger, for example, with fraud, the older adult experiences financial and psychological effects. In many cases, the older adult experiences serious physical consequences, deep psychological trauma, and loss of assets. These consequences affect the older adult not only on a personal level but also on an interpersonal level in his or her relationship with the perpetrator. When the perpetrator is a family member, the consequences can affect relationships with other family members and the abusive situation can be a source of major family discord. Family members may "take sides" or the abused older adult may be placed in a position of having to choose among dissenting family members. These conflicts often involve relationships among several generations and many sources (e.g., in-laws, partners, members of spouse's family from previous marriages). In situations involving a later life marriage, it is not unusual to encounter major disputes between the two "step families." These conflicts can be especially contentious in situations such as the following:

- When significant assets are required for long-term care of one or both of the parents and family members disagree about using resources
- When one or more of the family members perpetrate or support the abusive situations and others want to change it
- When family members want to protect their inheritance rather than allow the use of assets for care
- When family members have divisive power struggles related to decisions about care or finances

In some situations, two or more attorneys are involved, representing the older adult and several family members with conflicting interests. When the abuser is someone who provides care, resolution of the abusive situation can involve practical considerations related to the older adult's needs for care. Sometimes the resolution of abusive situations can entail decisions related to the older adult moving from a home setting to another, less desirable setting. Even when the home environment includes abusive relationships, the older adult may prefer that setting. Plans for resolving abusive situations can also involve major financial implications, which are based on the older adult's current financial assets as well as those that may have been jeopardized during an abusive situation.

When nurses encounter these kinds of situations, it is imperative that they advocate for the needs of the older adult and avoid showing partiality to any of those involved. In these situations, nurses have key roles in facilitating referrals for appropriate resources, such as social workers, mental health professionals, and adult protective services. It is also important to document any statements of the older adult or those who are involved and recognize that nursing documentation may provide crucial information related to the investigation and resolution of the situation. These situations usually involve psychological abuse and should be referred to adult protective services with the

CASE 10.3 Nurse Jonas Addresses Concerns About Family Dynamics

Nurse Jonas has been the primary care nurse for Mrs. Hickenbottom, who has been in the skilled rehabilitation unit for 2 weeks following a stroke. Mrs. Hickenbottom's son, Emmitt, lives with his mother and visits her every morning, often staying for a couple hours. During his visits, Emmitt makes a point of talking with Nurse Jonas about his mother's care and he is often highly critical of the staff. He repeatedly tells the staff that the care he provides at home is much better and "the sooner she gets out of this dump the better she will be." Mrs. Hickenbottom's two daughters visit in the afternoons and tell Nurse Jonas that their brother is unemployed and moved in with his mother after their father died 2 years ago. They have been concerned about her home situation, but they have not been able to visit for the last 6 months because Emmitt refuses to let them in. When they talk with their mother on the phone, she tells them that Emmitt is taking good care of her and that they do not need to bother coming over. The hospital records document that when Mrs. Hickenbottom was admitted with a stroke, her blood pressure was 220/135 and she was dehydrated.

When Nurse Jonas asks Mrs. Hickenbottom about her family, she says she is happy that Emmitt moved in because she was lonely and afraid to be alone after her husband died. She says, "Even though he has his problems, at least he is there for me." Nurse Jonas has overheard Emmitt talking with his mother and telling her that she does not need any more therapy and he can provide for her at home. He also says, "My sisters are jealous of me because I get to drive your car and live in the family home. They don't appreciate all I do for you and they are too busy with their husbands and kids to even visit you at home. The only reason they come to visit you here is to make the staff think they care about you. They just want to make sure you don't disinherit them." Later that day, Mrs. Hickenbottom tells Nurse Jonas that Emmitt plans to take her home tomorrow and they will "carry on just like we did before. We decided we don't want any of those therapists coming into our house." The next day, Emmitt packs his mother's belongings and assists her into his car. Mrs. Hickenbottom has signed her own discharge papers refusing any follow-up and stating that she understands she is qualified for skilled home care services but does not want them. Nurse Jonas calls adult protective services and requests an investigation.

expectation that the agency workers will advocate for the older adult's needs and at the same time respect his or her autonomy.

ADDRESSING LEGAL ISSUES

With the exception of reporting suspected abuse, legal issues related to individual elder abuse situations are beyond the scope of nursing. However, two nursing interventions are pertinent to addressing these issues. First, nurses can talk with older adults about advance directives that reflect their wishes if they are unable to make care-related decisions autonomously. Do not resuscitate (DNR) orders and similar legal documents are routinely addressed in health care settings, but it is important to recognize that other advance directives may be even more important in elder abuse situations. A durable power of attorney for health care is imperative because this document identifies a health care proxy who is responsible for health care decisions if the person is incapable of making those decisions independently. Nurses are in key positions to discuss advance directives with older adults, with emphasis on using these tools to better ensure that their wishes will be respected. This can be an important step in both preventing and addressing abuse, particularly in situations involving conflicts between the wishes of the older adult and those of family or among two or more family members. Institutional settings often have resources for addressing this as an aspect of advance directives, and nurses can initiate referrals for these resources.

Second, nurses can initiate referrals, or suggest that older adults and caregivers do so, to community-based resources that can address complex legal issues. For example, adult protective services agencies commonly provide consultation about legal issues, or resources for addressing these issues, even if the situation is not reportable as a suspected case. The national Eldercare Locator (www.eldercare.gov) provides information about all local aging services, including ones that address legal issues. Chapter 11 describes involuntary legal measures and community-based services that are specifically related to elder abuse situations.

KEY POINTS: WHAT NURSES NEED TO KNOW AND CAN DO

- Nursing interventions for elder abuse focus on reducing risks, addressing contributing conditions, managing consequences, and preventing further abuse.

- Building trust, establishing realistic goals, and addressing resistance are essential steps in addressing elder abuse situations.

- Nurses may need to address behavioral and mental issues that contribute to or are consequences of elder abuse situations (Box 10.1).

- Interventions that are more unique to elder abuse situations include teaching about self-protection and addressing risks to the safety of others.

- Elder abuse situations may involve issues related to family dynamics, legal considerations, and needs of caregivers.

- Nurses can use resources within health care settings to address issues related to elder abuse (Box 10.2).

- It is important to teach family caregivers about the following: appropriate care for managing health conditions of the dependent older adult, stress management related to the caregiving situation, and resources for education and support (Box 10.3).

REFERENCES

Anetzberger, G. J., Palmisano, B. R., Sanders, M., Bass, D., Dayton, C., Eckert, S., & Schimer, M. (2000). A model intervention for elder abuse and dementia. *Gerontologist, 40*, 492–497.

Cooper, C., & Livingston, G. (2014). Mental health/psychiatric issues in elder abuse and neglect. *Clinics in Geriatric Medicine, 30*, 839–850.

DuMont, J., Macdonald, S., Kosa, D., Elliot, S., Spencer, C., & Yaffe, M. (2015). Development of a comprehensive hospital-based elder abuse intervention: An initial systematic scoping review. *PLoS One, 10*(5), e0125105. doi:10.1371/journal.pone.0125105

Gelman, C. R., Sokoloff, T., Graziani, N., Arias, E., & Peralta, A. (2014). Individually-tailored support for ethnically-diverse caregivers: Enhancing our understanding of what is needed and what works. *Journal of Gerontological Social Work, 57*, 662–680.

Hirst, S. P., Penney, T., McNeill, S., Boscart, V. M., Podnieks, E., and Sinha, S. (2016). A systematic review to inform a best practice guideline on preventing and addressing abuse and neglect of older adults. *Canadian Journal on Aging, 35*(2), 242–260.

Mariam, L. M., McClure, R., Robinson, J. B., & Yang, J. A. (2015). Eliciting change in at-risk elders (ECARE): Evaluation of an elder abuse intervention program. *Journal of Elder Abuse & Neglect, 27*, 19–33.

Prochaska, J. O., & DiClemente, C. C. (1982). Stages and processes of self-change of smoking: Toward an integrative model of care. *Journal of Consulting and Clinical Psychology, 51*, 390–395.

Sirey, J. A., Berman, J., Salamone, A., Depasquale, A., Halkett, A., Raeifar, E., . . . Raue, P. J. (2015). Feasibility of integrating mental health screening and services into routine elder abuse practice to improve client outcomes. *Journal of Elder Abuse & Neglect, 27*, 254–269.

11

RESOURCES FOR ADDRESSING ELDER ABUSE

As discussed in Chapter 10, nurses have many opportunities to apply usual nursing interventions when they care for older adults who are in situations of actual or potential abuse. In addition to directly addressing these situations, nurses can often facilitate referrals for additional services and interventions that match the needs of their patients. Thus, nurses need to know not only about the range of services for elder abuse situations but also about how to access local resources. This chapter describes types of services that are commonly used to prevent and alleviate elder abuse situations in domestic settings and discusses ways in which nurses can facilitate use of these programs. Resources for addressing elder abuse in long-term care settings are discussed in Chapter 4, and Chapters 15 and 16 discuss resources for financial and sexual abuse, respectively.

GOALS AND TYPES OF SERVICES AND INTERVENTIONS

In health care settings, goals for care are limited in scope and necessarily focus on health-related needs of the older adult. In contrast, community-based services to address elder abuse focus on complex and long-term goals such as the following:

- Resolving crises and emergencies
- Ensuring victim safety

- Healing, empowering, and supporting victims
- Supporting the highest level of independence
- Preserving, protecting, and recovering assets
- Ensuring justice (Nurenberg, 2008)

Many types of community-based services are available to address these goals.

Types of services for elder abuse situations can be categorized according to their basic function as follows: core, emergency, support, rehabilitation, and prevention, as illustrated in Figure 11.1. Nurses in all settings can initiate or suggest referrals for services that are matched to types of abuse, as in the following examples:

- Self-neglect: home-delivered meals, community centers for meals and social activities, transportation, nonmedical home care services (e.g., companion, housekeeping, shopping, personal care)
- Neglect by caregivers: respite, care management, support and educational groups
- Physical abuse by trusted other: domestic violence hotlines
- Psychological abuse: counseling for older adult, mental health services for the older adult and perpetrator

Nurses in clinical settings have important roles in teaching about these resources because even when adult protective service workers are already involved, older adults may confide in and be amenable to suggestions from a nurse whom they trust. In many situations, nurses are the health care professionals who are best positioned to teach older adults and their families and caregivers about resources to alleviate risks for elder abuse.

AGING NETWORK SERVICES

The term *Aging Network* refers to the wide range of community-based services that are available through Area Agencies on Aging throughout the United States. Area Agencies on Aging were established in 1973 under the Older Americans Act to respond to the needs of Americans 60 years and over in every local community. In 2015, this Aging Network included 56 state agencies on aging, 629 area offices on aging, 246 Native American aging programs, about 29,000 service providers, and thousands of volunteers (Eldercare Locator, 2015). Virtually

FIGURE 11.1   Types of services needed by abused older adults and their caregivers.

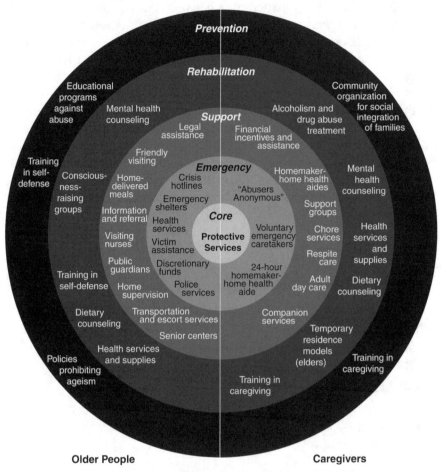

Reprinted by permission from Anetzberger (2010 [1982])

all Aging Networks address elder abuse in community settings through direct services, referrals, and cooperative working arrangements. Initially, these services were available only to older adults, but they have expanded to address the needs of adults with disabilities. In addition, they have increasingly addressed needs of caregivers by funding programs that provide respite, counseling, and education. Respite services, defined as any service whose primary goal is to relieve caregivers from usual caregiving responsibilities, are provided through community-based services such as nonmedical home care agencies, adult day centers, and assisted living facilities.

In addition to the many types of services that have been available for decades, a more recent focus that is particularly relevant to nurses is the development of partnerships between Area Agencies on Aging and health care systems to administer care transition programs to assist with discharges from acute care to home care settings. These programs have been funded by the Affordable Care Act to address concerns about unnecessary hospitalizations of older adults. Another focus related to health care for older adults with chronic conditions is the provision of evidence-based health promotion programs endorsed by the Centers for Disease Control and Prevention and the Administration on Aging. Nurses can encourage older adults or their caregivers to explore these types of resources, which are described in Box 11.1. In many situations, services such as these are effective in reducing risk for abuse and alleviating contributing conditions when abuse is occurring or has occurred.

BOX 11.1 Services Provided by Aging Networks

Services most commonly available
- Meals, in congregate settings or delivered to homes
- Chore services: housekeeping, shopping
- Assistance with personal care
- Transportation
- Socialization in community centers
- Adult day centers

Services to address needs of caregivers
- Respite
- Caregiver education
- Counseling
- Support groups

Services to divert people from prematurely being admitted to a long-term care setting
- Assessment
- Counseling about options

(continued)

BOX 11.1 Services Provided by Aging Networks *(continued)*

- Arrangement for and supervision of home care service
- Care management and coordination
- Caregiver education

Services to ease the transition from an institutional setting to home

- Caregiver education to help prepare for the person's return to home
- Coaching for older adults and caregivers
- Teaching about health conditions
- Provision of or payment for home modifications

Evidence-based health promotion programs

- Self-management of chronic disease
- Diabetes self-management
- Fall prevention education

ACCESS TO SERVICES

Services delineated in Box 11.1 are generally available according to geographic location with additional criteria applying in some cases. For example, some programs are based on assessment of need, such as being homebound to qualify for home-delivered meals. Services are sometimes provided without charge; in other cases, fees may be based on income or other criteria. The Eldercare Locator is an essential national resource for information about all services within the Aging Network. Online information for types of services by geographic location is available at www.eldercare.gov. During weekday business hours, information specialists are available at 1-800-677-1116 to discuss programs and services in English or Spanish or with a telecommunication device for people who are deaf. In addition, online chats or language interpretation services are available for 150 languages during these hours. In 2014, 27% of the calls were related to elder abuse and 29% addressed caregiver issues (Administration for Community Living, 2014).

CASE 11.1 Elder Network Services for Mrs. Kryzynski

Mrs. Kryzynski, who is 85 years old and lives in her own home, was admitted to the hospital 2 days ago with fractured ribs, neck pain, and multiple contusions over her chest and face. While driving to church, she had been rear-ended after stopping suddenly—and unnecessarily—at a yellow caution light. The emergency department physician admitted her because, in addition to her injuries, her breathing was labored and her lungs were congested. Chronic conditions include diabetes, hypertension, rheumatoid arthritis, macular degeneration, and chronic obstructive pulmonary disease.

During her hospitalization, Mrs. Kryzynski confided that she is reluctant to drive again because she has had several "close calls" even before the accident 2 days ago. She states, "My eyesight has been getting a little worse every few months but if I can't drive I'm afraid I'll become a recluse like my friend who died a couple months ago." Now her car is damaged again and she indicates that she will give up driving rather than get her car repaired. She also tells you that she needs to drive to the grocery store at least every week and she definitely does not want to give up her attendance at church. When you review the discharge orders with Mrs. Kryzynski, you add information about calling the Eldercare Locator to find resources for transportation. You also suggest that she may want to consider attending the local senior center for lunches and social activities, so she does not become socially isolated.

RESOURCES FOR SPECIFIC GROUPS

In addition to services commonly included in the Aging Network, faith-based and culturally specific resources may be available in some communities. Also, the Veterans Administration is often overlooked as a resource for older adults and caregivers. Older adults who identify with a particular group or religious denomination may find that these resources are more acceptable than other community-based organizations. Nurses can also consider suggesting resources such as Alcoholics Anonymous or Al-Anon in situations involving substance abuse by either the older adult or a family caregiver. Local offices on aging can usually provide information about programs such as the types described in this section.

Faith community nursing (also called parish nursing), which has been recognized by the American Nurses Association since 1998, is a specialized practice of professional nursing that focuses on care of the spirit as well as on the prevention or minimization of illness within the context of a faith community (American Nurses Association, 2012). Faith community nurses spend 50% to 100% of their time providing services to older adults, such as referrals, personal counseling, spiritual support, and health advocacy (King & Pappas-Rogich, 2011). Many Jewish organizations provide a wide range of community-based services for older adults, including programs specifically addressing elder abuse. These resources may be particularly effective for addressing issues related to caregivers or family dynamics and situations in which the older adult would benefit from advocacy.

Culturally specific resources are increasingly available, as discussed in Chapter 5. Since 1978, the Older Americans Act has funded Aging Network services for Indian tribal organizations, with a current focus of these programs on elder abuse. Culturally specific programs are especially pertinent for older adults who are immigrants and for those who do not speak English. In recent years, there has been increasing development of services for Korean or Chinese older adults, including community centers, home care services, adult day centers, and options for long-term care.

The Veterans Administration provides many home and community-based services for veterans of any age and their caregivers. Services that are relevant to prevention of elder abuse include home-based primary care, homemaker and home health aide services, respite care, care management, rehabilitation therapies, and adult day health care. Older adults who are veterans are often unaware of home and community-based services, particularly if they receive their primary care from sources not connected with the Veterans Administration. Nurses can encourage veterans and their family caregivers to explore resources for home and community-based services at www.caregiver.va.gov.

COMPREHENSIVE GERIATRIC ASSESSMENT PROGRAMS

Comprehensive geriatric assessment programs are a resource within the health care system that can be used for addressing many situations involving actual or potential abuse, particularly those that involve questions about the health, functioning, and decision-making capacity of the older adult or plans for long-term care. Comprehensive geriatric assessment programs provide multidimensional and multidisciplinary

CASE 11.2 Mr. Hobbs, World War II Veteran

Mr. Hobbs was hospitalized several years ago with a blood clot in his leg. Upon returning home, Mr. Hobbs had limited mobility and his wife had a difficult time transferring him between his bed and his lift chair. The Veterans Administration hospital provided a Hoyer lift, which enabled Mrs. Hobbs to continue caring for her husband in their home. Two-and-a-half years ago, Mr. Hobbs was admitted into the home-based primary care program for monthly blood draws. Over time, home-based primary care provided additional medical equipment, including a hospital bed, electric scooter, and an exercise peddler. Mrs. Hobbs was a devoted caregiver and did not want to use the services of the homemaker and home health aide or respite programs. Mrs. Hobbs continued to care for her husband all alone, even sacrificing her health at times. During monthly visits, the home-based primary care nurse and social worker would reinforce the programs available and encourage Mrs. Hobbs to use them to decrease some of the work she did on a daily basis. Eventually, Mr. and Mrs. Hobbs began to accept additional services. Now a home health aide assists Mr. Hobbs with bathing, grooming, dressing, and transfers. Mrs. Hobbs agreed to use the in-home respite program, and now says, "I didn't realize that just to get away really does help." Mrs. Hobbs describes a recent time when she was recovering from an illness and used the in-home respite program. While she was resting, the home health aide cleaned her home, which is still something she never expects but truly appreciates.

Adapted from *Donetta's Story*, posted at www.caregiver.va.gov

assessments of all aspects of health and functioning and recommend interventions to help the older adult function at his or her highest level. Assessments are performed and discussed by team members, which typically include geriatricians, gerontological nurses, social workers, geriatric mental health professionals, and rehabilitation therapists. Team members assess the older adult and seek input from family members and caregivers. The team recommends interventions to address issues and works with older adults and caregivers to develop a plan for the appropriate level of care in home, community-based, or long-term care settings.

Outpatient geriatric assessment programs are widely available at large medical centers, teaching hospitals, and university-based gerontology centers. Inpatient geriatric assessment programs are also available either as a specialized geriatric unit or as a component of geriatric behavior and mental health services. Geriatric assessment programs generally accept referrals from any source and serve as consultants for primary care providers on an intermittent or short-term basis. Nurses in all settings can teach older adults and family caregivers about these resources whenever questions arise about decision-making capacity or the most appropriate level of care for an older adult.

CASE 11.3 Miryam Perlman, Geriatric Assessment Program

At Miryam Perlman's 80th birthday party, her family and friends toasted her long-standing characteristics of being "feisty and independent to the end." During the 8 months since her party, however, more than a few people who have seen her recently have noticed that her fastidious way of being well groomed and neatly dressed has changed. Her clothes are soiled and hang loosely. Several months ago, she stopped attending the Shabbat services at the Beth Israel Temple, which she had attended for many decades. After members of the congregation expressed their concerns to Rabbi Cohen, he visited Miryam and was troubled by what he observed. Miryam's house was in disarray, with dirty dishes piled in the kitchen, and little evidence of proper food preparation. He guessed that she had not bathed in quite a while and her hair was oily and uncombed. When he talked about recent events at the Temple, she conversed as if she knew about them, but the details she described were related to events that happened 20 years ago. When he asked about visits from her son or daughter, who both live in other states, she said, "Oh, they were here just a few days ago, and they are fine." He asked if it would be OK if he called her daughter, and, although she saw no need for the contact, Miryam agreed.

When Rabbi Cohen talked with Miryam's daughter, she told him that neither she nor her brother had seen their mother since Miryam's birthday party 8 months ago. They have both talked with their mother on the phone, and expressed their concerns that she seems a "little fuzzy" but she always insists that "everything is just fine here."

(continued)

CASE 11.3 Miryam Perlman, Geriatric Assessment Program
(continued)

After talking with Rabbi Cohen about her mother's situation, Miryam's daughter, Adina, finds information about the Mt. Sinai geriatric assessment program and makes an appointment to accompany her mother for the assessment.

When Adina takes Miryam to the assessment program, the social worker spends time with Adina while the gerontological clinical nurse specialist, a geriatrician, and an occupational therapist assess Miryam. The professionals share their findings in a team meeting, and then sit with Adina and Miryam to review the findings and make recommendations. The geriatrician reports that the likely diagnosis for Miryam is mild cognitive impairment, but further tests will identify or rule out medical factors that should be addressed. Team goals are to recommend interventions that will prevent the situation from developing into self-neglect and to support Miryam's highest level of functioning. In the interim, the team recommends that a care manager from the local Jewish Family Services program meets with Adina and Miryam while Adina is still in town. The care manager will work with Miryam to gain acceptance of in-home services, such as housekeeping and assistance with shopping and personal care. She will also maintain phone and e-mail contact with Adina and accompany Miryam to follow-up appointments at the geriatric assessment program.

SERVICES TO ADDRESS NEEDS OF CAREGIVERS

Nurses commonly have frequent contact with family caregivers and are in key positions to discuss community-based resources. This is particularly important for families and caregivers of people with dementia because of the increased risk for elder abuse in these situations. In addition to the Aging Network services that address needs of caregivers, many resources are available for education, support, and actual caregiving. Local Alzheimer's Associations are a primary source of information about services to address caregiver needs, and the information is applicable to all caregiving situations regardless of medical diagnoses. Box 11.2 lists governmental and nonprofit resources to support caregivers.

> **BOX 11.2 Resources to Support Caregivers**
>
> Alzheimer's Association, www.alz.org
> Caregiver Action Network, www.caregiveraction.org
> Eldercare Locator, www.eldercare.gov
> Family Caregiver Alliance, www.caregiver.org
> National Alliance for Caregiving, www.caregiving.org
> National Center on Elder Abuse, www.ncea.aoa.gov
> National Respite Network and Resource Center, www.archrespite.org
> Rosalyn Carter Institute for Caregiving, www.rosalynncarter.org
> Veterans Administration Caregiver Support, www.caregiver.va.gov

RESOURCES SPECIFICALLY FOR ELDER ABUSE

Resources described in this section are used to resolve actual elder abuse situations and generally are accessed through public agencies, such as adult protective services. Although nurses are usually not involved with referrals for these programs, nurses are often in positions of teaching older adults and families about the scope of community-based resources for addressing abuse.

Adult Protective Service Agencies

In addition to investigating alleged elder abuse cases (discussed in Chapter 6), adult protective service agencies provide interventions when the older adult is willing to accept services. If case workers assess that services are necessary but the older adult refuses to accept them, the adult protective services agency may arrange for an evaluation of the person's decision-making capacity. If a court deems that the person is incompetent, legal actions are initiated, but in all other situations the person's autonomy will be respected.

Care management and care coordination are essential components of adult protective service agencies. Agencies are staffed by several levels and types of workers, including nurses, social workers, and nonmedical home care assistance. In addition, they are an integral part of the Aging Network and commonly have contractual arrangements with other professionals and agencies, such as psychiatric and mental health services, legal advisors, and animal protection agencies. Public health and home care agencies often provide nursing consultations, assessment, or direct care interventions for adult protective agencies that do not employ nurses. Case consultation is a service offered by adult protective service agencies that is especially relevant to nurses who are seeking guidance about a questionable situation that they encounter in their clinical setting.

Multidisciplinary Teams

Since the early 2000s, multidisciplinary teams (also called M-teams, interdisciplinary teams, or I-teams) have been considered the "gold standard" for addressing elder abuse. Teams generally include professionals who offer the perspectives of law, nursing, medicine, psychiatry, social work, and rehabilitation therapy, with additional disciplines included when required. When legal interventions are being considered, the multidisciplinary team conducts or arranges for a comprehensive assessment, including all aspects of the person's functioning and decision-making capacity, the involvement of the family and significant others in meeting basic needs, and the ability of the older person to participate in developing a safe and realistic plan of action.

Roles and activities of multidisciplinary teams vary, but an overarching goal is to provide a holistic perspective, which is essential for thoroughly assessing the problem and determining appropriate solutions. In addition, team members collaborate in handling complex and difficult cases and they can establish effective approaches to elder abuse prevention and treatment (Anetzberger, 2011). Multidisciplinary teams differ in their ability or willingness to provide direct interventions; however, the case review from knowledgeable professionals is a valuable resource for the service providers who are responsible for interventions.

Nurses participate in these teams and provide initial and ongoing assessment as well as direct care or consultation related to health-related issues, such as management of medical conditions, treatment of pressure ulcers, and education about safety risks. Chapter 13 illustrates the way in which a multidisciplinary team provides consultation to a nurse to address self-neglect in a rural setting.

Specialized Elder Abuse Teams

In recent years, specialized teams have evolved to address particular elder abuse situations, such as financial abuse (discussed in Chapter 15) and hoarding, including animal hoarding. Elder abuse forensic centers provide multidisciplinary case reviews of situations that involve possible violations of laws (e.g., financial abuse, physical abuse, sexual abuse). Box 11.3 describes examples of specialized elder abuse teams and services.

BOX 11.3 Examples of Specialized Elder Abuse Teams and Services

Elder Abuse Forensic Center
- Multiagency team case review and development of action plan
- Medical and neuropsychological evaluations
- Forensic evaluation and documentation
- Victim assistance and support services
- Consultation, education, and training

Texas Elder Abuse and Mistreatment (TEAM)
- Medical evaluations in homes, hospital, or outpatient settings
- Teleconsulting: provides offsite medical consultation to adult protective service workers
- Financial abuse specialist team (FAST): includes medical professionals and law enforcement members who review cases of exploitation and fraud committed against the elderly
- Elder abuse fatality review team: reviews suspicious elder deaths
- Resource rooms: enable adult protective services workers to find basic necessities and emergency supplies, such as dietary supplements, adult diapers, and assistive devices

Elder Abuse Institute of Maine
- Martha's Cottage: provides transitional home for elder abuse victims, who can stay for up to 24 months

Fatality (Death) Review Teams
- Multidisciplinary teams: explore unexplained deaths of older adults, distinguish "natural" deaths from those associated with crimes, and shed light on events leading up to deaths
- Assist in prosecution of alleged perpetrator

Emergency Shelter and Transitional Housing Programs

Emergency shelter programs provide a safe place where abused older adults can receive immediate and short-term health, housing, legal, and counseling services. These programs are usually located in long-term care settings, such as nursing homes or assisted living facilities. The Weinberg Center for Elder Abuse Prevention, which is part of the New York City Hebrew Home, established the first emergency shelter program for older adults in 2005. Since then, shelters specifically for older adults have been developed in many states, including Arizona, Minnesota, Nebraska, Ohio, and Vermont. In 2009, the Elder Abuse Institute of Maine opened the first transitional home for victims of elder abuse, called Martha's Cottage, with initial and ongoing funding from the U.S. Department of Justice. Women age 60 and older who are seeking safety from a violent household can stay in the house for up to 24 months.

Nurses in emergency departments and outpatient settings can initiate referrals or teach older adults about these resources. In hospital settings, information about emergency shelters can be included in discharge instructions for older adults who are choosing to return to situations of domestic abuse. It is important to maintain strict confidentiality about this information and assure that perpetrators do not become aware of it. Information about local emergency shelters is available at the National Domestic Violence Hotline (1-800-799-7223 [SAFE]) or through the adult protective service agencies listed in Appendix B.

CASE 11.4 Emergency Shelter for Mrs. Ackerman

During a follow-up appointment for hypertension, Nurse Practitioner Laura notes that Mrs. Ackerman seems unusually anxious and has black and blue bruises across her forehead, around her left eye, and on both upper arms. Mrs. Ackerman is 73 years old and lives with her husband, who is 67 years old. When Nurse Practitioner Laura asks her patient about the bruises, Mrs. Ackerman initially says she walked into the door when she got up to go to the bathroom a couple nights ago. Mrs. Ackerman avoids eye contact and changes the subject after answering briefly. When Nurse Practitioner Laura asks her patient if she feels safe at home, Mrs. Ackerman begins to cry and admits that her husband grabbed her by her arms and threw her

(continued)

> **CASE 11.4 Emergency Shelter for Mrs. Ackerman (continued)**
>
> into a dresser in their bedroom when he was drunk. Although he has threatened her in the past, she now has difficulty getting away because the arthritis in her knees interferes with her mobility. Mrs. Ackerman says she is afraid to return home because when she left earlier that day he was at a bar with his friends. Nurse Practitioner Laura reports the situation to adult protective services and also arranges for Mrs. Ackerman to be admitted to the emergency shelter program at the local continuing care center.

INVOLUNTARY MEASURES

Although the first principle of adult protective services is to protect the person's autonomy, some situations involve the use of involuntary measures, such as guardianship or civil commitment. State laws define the processes for these measures, which are implemented under court supervision. Nurses in most health care settings are not directly involved with involuntary interventions, but it is important to be aware of these interventions when caring for older adults in abusive or potentially abusive situations. When nurses address any situations involving consideration of involuntary measures, they can call adult protective services. They also have roles in explaining these measures to families.

Guardianship (also called conservatorship) is the legal process that appoints a surrogate decision maker for people who have been determined to be incompetent (i.e., unable to make decisions for themselves). Court proceedings can be initiated by any concerned individual, including families, health care providers, attorneys, or adult protective service agencies. The person is entitled to legal representation and an extensive evaluation is required. If the judge determines that the person is incompetent, a partial or full guardianship is appointed. Although guardianships can be revoked or reversed through additional court action, it generally remains in place until the incompetent person dies. Usually, guardianship is initiated only as a last resort when no other legal intervention is appropriate because it is a drastic measure that takes away rights and entails court proceedings and ongoing court monitoring.

Civil commitment, also known as an involuntary psychiatric hospitalization, is used when older adults are too impaired to protect themselves or when they pose a threat to themselves or others. Gero-psychiatric programs and geriatric behavioral health units in hospitals accept involuntary admissions for evaluation, management, and discharge planning.

KEY POINTS: WHAT NURSES NEED TO KNOW AND CAN DO

- Many community-based resources are available for preventing and addressing elder abuse.

- Community-based services for abused older adults focus on complex and long-term goals, including supporting the older adult's highest level of independence.

- Community-based services address the needs of caregivers as well as of older adults.

- Recognize that specialized programs and services for specific groups may be acceptable even when other programs are not.

- It is imperative to build on a trusting nurse–patient relationship to address barriers to the use of services.

- Nurses have important roles in teaching older adults and their caregivers about accessing needed services.

REFERENCES

Administration for Community Living. (2014). *Eldercare Locator Data Report.* Washington, DC: U.S. Department of Health and Human Services, Administration for Community Living.

American Nurses Association. (2012). *Faith community nursing: Scope and standards of practice.* Silver Spring, MD: American Nurses Association.

Anetzberger, G. J. (2010[1982]). *Report of the Elder Abuse Project: Recommendations for addressing the problem of elder abuse in Cuyahoga County.* Cleveland, OH: Federation for Community Planning.

Anetzberger, G. J. (2011). The evolution of an interdisciplinary response to elder abuse. *Marquette Elder's Advisor, 13*(1), 107–128.

Eldercare Locator. (2015). *The Aging Network.* Retrieved at www.eldercare.gov

King, M. A., & Pappas-Rogich, M. (2011). Faith community nurses: Implementing *Healthy People* standards to promote the health of elderly clients. *Geriatric Nursing, 32,* 459–464.

Nurenberg, L. (2008). Preventing and treating elder abuse. In L. Nurenberg (Ed.), *Elder abuse prevention: Emerging trends and promising strategies* (pp. 101–143). New York, NY: Springer Publishing Company.

NURSES IN ACTION ADDRESSING ELDER ABUSE IN CLINICAL SETTINGS

NURSES IN ACTION ADDRESSING DOMESTIC ELDER ABUSE ACROSS SETTINGS

This chapter describes the case of Joseph and Sophie Peterson as it "unfolds" across various settings to illustrate how nurses in acute care and home care settings work with other professionals to resolve a domestic elder abuse situation. As the case unfolds, nurses use their assessment and intervention skills to identify and address risks for and consequences of elder abuse during different phases. The case is a composite of this author's experiences in clinical settings.

OVERVIEW: JOSEPH AND SOPHIE PETERSON

Joseph and Sophie Peterson have been married for 49 years and describe themselves as having "many ups and downs through the years but always making it through together." Eight years ago, at the age of 67, Joseph retired from his long-term career as vice president of a major manufacturing business. Joseph and Sophie's four children are married with families, but they all live several states away and visit primarily on holidays. Sophie attends weekly services at the nearby Catholic Church and also volunteers at the church as a member of the Altar & Rosary Society. Four years ago, Joseph had coronary artery bypass surgery after a serious myocardial infarction. After being discharged from the hospital, Joseph participated in a cardiac rehabilitation program, but after a few weeks he showed no motivation to continue with healthy behaviors. After he stopped going to cardiac rehabilitation, Joseph began spending more and more time away from home playing cards with his "poker buddies" until he was getting together with them almost daily. Although he had quit smoking cigarettes when he had the bypass surgery, he began smoking cigars whenever he was with his poker buddies. Of course, beer and chips were routinely consumed during the card games.

Although Sophie was concerned about her husband's sedentary lifestyle and the amount of time he spent away from home, she was even more concerned about the way in which Joseph was treating her when he was at home. Sophie thought she was tactful when she tried to talk with him about these changes, but she soon realized that no matter how she approached the topic of his health, he became angry and defensive. A couple years ago, Joseph started grabbing Sophie's arms and shaking her when she expressed concerns about his health. His usual verbal response was, "I'm old enough to take care of my own health and you should just worry about how fat you're getting." Sophie never told anyone about these episodes and she focused on developing an attitude of acceptance, even as she observed that his health was declining. She found great solace in her faith community and began going to church daily.

Joseph's health continued to deteriorate but he refused to go to medical appointments until his breathing became so limited that he had difficulty getting to the card games. Sophie's concerns escalated, not only about her husband's physical limitations, but also about the changes in his personality. Even when Sophie was particularly careful about the way she talked to Joseph, she frequently had to protect herself from his verbal abuse. When Sophie felt physically threatened by his behaviors, she could protect herself by quickly moving out of his way because he had difficulty breathing when he exerted himself or tried to get out of his chair. As long as Sophie was alert to potential threats she was safe, but sometimes she did not move quickly enough and Joseph grabbed her and left bruises on both her arms.

On July 20, Joseph fell while trying to get out of his reclining chair and he was unable to get up from the floor. Despite Joseph's protests, Sophie called 911 and the emergency medical attendants insisted that they transport him to the hospital, with Sophie accompanying him in the ambulance.

UNFOLDING CASE PART ONE: NURSE CYNTHIA AT WELLSFORD COMMUNITY HOSPITAL, EMERGENCY DEPARTMENT, JULY 20

What Nurse Cynthia Knows

Joseph Peterson is a 75-year-old male brought to the emergency department for evaluation of dyspnea and falling. The bed is in the high-Fowler's position and the patient is receiving oxygen at 2 L per nasal cannula.

Nurse Cynthia documents the following pertinent assessment findings:

Height:	5'10"
Weight:	218 lbs.
Temperature:	98.4°
Pulse:	112, irregular
Respirations:	24
Pulse oximeter:	91%
Blood pressure:	176/102

3+ edema and dark red discoloration of both feet, extending to knees

Blue-colored bruise on left posterior thigh, irregular oval shaped, measuring 5 cm by 8 cm, reportedly from hitting leg against a small table when patient fell from chair earlier today

Adventitious sounds throughout both lungs

Although Joseph is socially appropriate to the staff in the ED, he frequently yells at his wife, especially if she tries to offer any information about his medical care. For example, when Sophie tried to offer information about Joseph sleeping in the recliner chair most nights because he was having trouble getting upstairs to their bedroom, Joseph angrily said, "You stay out of this, Sophie, I can talk for myself." Sophie sits in a chair as far from Joseph as is physically possible in the small ED cubicle and she seems to be intimidated by him.

What Nurse Cynthia Thinks

When I was leaving the room to call Dr. Thomas, Sophie followed me and asked if I had a minute to talk with her. She told me that she was concerned about her husband not going to doctor appointments and not getting his medications refilled since the last year. Sophie also said that he has become forgetful and gets very angry and upset if she raises any questions about his health. When Sophie asked if her husband could be evaluated for "old timers' disease and memory problems," she was on the verge of tears but was very stoic. I'm sure that Sophie wanted to talk more, but when Joseph yelled loudly for her to come back in the room, she abruptly stopped our conversation and returned to her husband's bedside. I noted that both of Sophie's lower arms had multiple bruises, ranging in color from yellow to purple, but I didn't have a chance to ask her about the bruises or about any concerns for herself. The bruises on both of Sophie's lower arms looked like the kind that are associated with being grabbed. Based on what I know about elder abuse, I wonder if Joseph could be abusing Sophie, and I have questions about Joseph's mental status, as well as self-neglect for not following through with necessary medical care.

What Nurse Cynthia Does

Nurse Cynthia documents that Mrs. Peterson reported concerns about her husband's difficult behaviors, along with a request for further evaluation of his memory. She also adds the nursing diagnosis of Self-Neglect on Joseph's chart as an impetus for further evaluation of Joseph's mental status and their home situation. In addition, she discusses her concerns with the attending doctor, who responds that he will make a referral for social services when Joseph is admitted for heart failure and order a consult for an evaluation of his mental status.

UNFOLDING CASE PART TWO: NURSE SHAWNA AT WELLSFORD COMMUNITY HOSPITAL, UNIT 2C, JULY 24

What Nurse Shawna Knows

As the geriatric resource nurse at Wellsford Community Hospital, Nurse Shawna is available for consultations to nursing staff who request her services based on concerns about a geriatric patient with complex needs. Several staff nurses have documented concerns not only about Joseph Peterson's ability to adhere to a medical treatment plan after discharge but also about his interactions with his wife. Nurse Shawna reviews Joseph's chart and notes the following pertinent information:

> Patient was admitted with unstable heart failure most likely associated with nonadherence to prescribed medications during the

past several years. Psychiatry consultation documents new diagnosis of dementia, based on comprehensive evaluation of mental status and medical conditions. A physical therapy evaluation was performed yesterday because Joseph has not been walking and he has refused to get out of bed, except when he goes to the bathroom with two nurses assisting him. Medical and psychiatry notes document that the patient reports "occasional alcohol use in social settings," but the social service note states that Mrs. Peterson reports that the patient drinks at least four beers when he is with his poker buddies, which is an almost daily occurrence.

Staff nurses document that Mrs. Peterson visits daily and the patient often raises his voice and is very demanding with his wife. Moreover, when she wants to leave he yells and loudly tells her that she needs to sit quietly by his bedside in case he needs anything. Several nursing notes document that Mrs. Peterson has talked to the nurses out of the patient's hearing and she has expressed concerns about her husband's behaviors, especially after he returns home from his poker games. Nursing notes also document that Mrs. Peterson seems anxious and overwhelmed and has expressed concerns about being able to care for her husband when he returns home. A social service worker met with the patient and his wife separately, and Mrs. Peterson is receptive to services for home care; however, the patient refuses to allow any help in their home and Mrs. Peterson states that she will do whatever her husband wants.

What Nurse Shawna Does

Nurse Shawna visits Joseph Peterson while his wife is at his bedside and tells them that she is working with the doctors and hospital staff to develop a plan for Joseph to return home with help. Joseph adamantly states that they do not need any help and that his wife is perfectly capable of taking care of his needs. When Nurse Shawna points out that he would qualify for home-based physical therapy because he requires two nurses to assist him getting out of bed, he says, "I'm perfectly comfortable staying in bed and when I feel like getting up I will. Sophie can help me if I need it." Nurse Shawna suggests that a visiting nurse would also review his medications and check his heart and lungs to see if his heart condition remains stable. In addition, there will be an order for oxygen at home and the visiting nurse can make sure Mr. and Mrs. Peterson know how to use the equipment. Again, Mr. Peterson adamantly states that his wife can take care of anything he needs. He then states, "And we don't need any of your advice either, so there's nothing more to discuss."

Later, when Nurse Shawna is at the nursing station, she notices that Mrs. Peterson has come out of her husband's room looking for her. Sophie says that she told her husband she was going to the cafeteria for lunch but, in reality, she is hoping to have time to talk with Nurse Shawna in private. In a conference room, Nurse Shawna obtains the following information from Sophie:

> Sophie tearfully reports that no matter what she has tried to do to influence her husband toward healthy behaviors, she has failed to do so. He has refused to see any doctors for almost two years and he usually took only half of his medications so they would last longer. He has not been able to get refills for at least six months because his doctors won't write the prescriptions without seeing him. He usually took his medications for a few days prior to family visits, so his feet would not be swollen. Yesterday after the consulting psychiatrist told them that Joseph had dementia, Joseph said, "That doctor doesn't know what he's talking about. If I had dementia, I wouldn't be winning all those poker games. I don't believe a word he said, and he's not my regular doctor anyway so we don't have to pay any attention to him. When I get home, everything will be OK, just like it used to be."
>
> When Nurse Shawna asked about Joseph's consumption of alcohol, Sophie said that he smells of beer and cigar smoke when he comes home, but he gets angry if she asks anything about what they do at the poker games, so she doesn't ask any questions. When their sons come to visit on holidays, they drink beer and scotch while they watch sports on television, but Joseph does not drink in front of Sophie. When Nurse Shawna asks if Joseph has ever harmed her, Sophie says, "He can't get to me anymore now that he's in bed and I know that I can get out of his way when I need to."

Nurse Shawna would like to spend more time talking with Sophie, but after 15 minutes, Sophie says she needs to get back in the room or Joseph will yell at her for being gone so long and he may suspect she is talking with someone about him.

What Nurse Shawna Thinks

I am concerned about the risk of abuse in this situation. If Sophie feels safer when Joseph is physically limited, she may not want him to regain his independence and that certainly will influence his care. It's difficult for me to obtain more information from Sophie, but the social worker can call Sophie at her home and make an appointment to talk with her before she visits Joseph tomorrow. As a nurse, I can focus on Sophie's role as a caregiver for Joseph and make sure there is follow-up on my concerns. My priority is to focus on a discharge plan for Joseph so there's follow-up on his care. Probably his resistance to home care is associated with him wanting to maintain the lifestyle he has, but we need to find a way to get him to accept a visiting nurse.

What Nurse Shawna Does

Nurse Shawna discusses her concerns with the attending physician, who says he will tell Joseph that home care is required unless Joseph wants to go to a nursing facility for therapy until he can be safely cared for at home. Nurse Shawna advises the nursing staff to talk with Joseph about accepting the referral for physical therapy and skilled nursing as an essential part of the plan for him to regain his independence.

UNFOLDING CASE, PART THREE: NURSE ROGER AT WELLSFORD VISITING NURSE ASSOCIATION, JULY 28
What Nurse Roger Knows

Nurse Roger visits the Petersons to provide skilled nursing after Joseph was discharged to home yesterday with diagnoses of heart failure and dementia. Nurse Roger notes that the house is cluttered, musty smelling, and in need of cleaning. Sophie greets Nurse Roger and accompanies him upstairs to the bedroom where Joseph is confined to bed. The oxygen equipment is sitting unplugged in a corner of the room and the smell of a recently smoked cigar provides a clue about the reason that Joseph is not using oxygen. The only nursing assessment findings that are not within normal range are pulse oximeter of 87%, respirations 24, and adventitious sounds in both lungs. While Nurse Roger assesses Joseph and begins documenting his assessment findings in the electronic medical record on his laptop, Joseph angrily and impatiently says, "Do you have to do all that computer stuff right now? Can't you see I'm exhausted and can't deal with this nonsense? I think your job here is done. We're getting along fine without you coming in here anyway. You can leave now and don't bother coming back." Although

Nurse Roger is unable to review the medications with either Mr. or Mrs. Peterson, he does observe written prescriptions among the discharge papers on the dresser. When he asks about the medications, Sophie says her husband would not let her get the new prescriptions filled because they still had medicines left from before.

Joseph then tells Sophie to show Nurse Roger the way out of the house. Sophie walks downstairs with Nurse Roger and begins whispering that she does not know what to do because her husband will not listen to anyone and he just wants to stay in his bed and watch television. Joseph's friends plan to visit tomorrow and she knows they will bring him beer and cigars. As Sophie is whispering her concerns to Nurse Roger, Joseph yells for her to get back upstairs and bring him some water, then she quickly escorts Nurse Roger to the door and tells him he probably should not return.

What Nurse Roger Thinks

I am very concerned about this situation and I doubt that Mr. Peterson is taking his pills now, because the discharge summary documents a history of nonadherence and concerns about potential self-neglect. When I asked about reviewing Joseph's medications, he became very anxious. Even though I usually use my laptop to enter the assessment information during my visit, next time I will take a few notes while I'm with Mr. Peterson and enter the information for his chart after I leave the house because this seemed to upset him. I need to establish a relationship with Mr. Peterson and find some common ground so I can continue my visits for skilled care, which he certainly needs. My primary goal at this time is to gain acceptance so I can continue working with this situation.

What Nurse Roger Does

As Nurse Roger is leaving the house, he quietly asks Sophie about a time he can call and talk with her. Sophie says that her husband will be sleeping late tomorrow morning and she says she will call Nurse Roger around 9 a.m. so her husband will not hear the phone ring. On July 29, when Sophie calls Nurse Roger she confides that her husband does not want anyone to know that he smoked cigars and drank beer and he wants her to "wait on him hand and foot." He is content to stay in his room, as long as his friends come and play cards there.

Moreover, he says he will not use the oxygen because he does not like being "attached to a cord" and he can breathe well enough as long as he does not get out of bed. When Nurse Roger discusses the order for a physical therapy service to help Joseph regain his mobility, Sophie says they do not need any therapist coming in because her husband will not cooperate anyway. When Nurse Roger suggests that a home health aide could come to assist with Joseph's care, Sophie says, "I'm the only one he will let touch him and we are managing just fine." Sophie then tells Nurse Roger that she cannot stay on the phone because Joseph is yelling for her to come upstairs. Nurse Roger tells Sophie that he will plan to come again tomorrow at 9:30 a.m.

Nurse Roger visits on July 30 at 9:30 a.m. but finds the Peterson house closed up with curtains drawn on all the windows. The car is in the driveway and the dog is in the fenced-in back yard, but Sophie does not answer the door. When Nurse Roger calls on his cell phone from the driveway, the phone rings but goes unanswered. Nurse Roger makes several more phone calls over the next few days but is unable to make contact. On August 8, Nurse Roger reviews the case with his supervisor and then makes a report to the local adult protective services agency.

UNFOLDING CASE PART FOUR: NURSE ROGER WORKS WITH PROTECTIVE SERVICES SOCIAL WORKER TO ADDRESS DOMESTIC ELDER ABUSE

What Nurse Roger Knows

On August 12, the county adult protective services worker, Ms. McConnell, calls Nurse Roger and reports that Mrs. Peterson opened the door yesterday and the social worker found Mrs. Peterson very distraught about her husband not being able to breathe. Mrs. Peterson told Ms. McConnell that she wanted to let the visiting nurse come back last week but her husband had yelled and screamed so much that she was afraid of what he would do if she let anyone in. Mrs. Peterson said that her husband refused to take any pills and would not use his oxygen, even though she told him he would feel better. Mr. Peterson was having difficulty breathing and his legs were so swollen that he could not get out of bed, which was wet with urine. Ms. McConnell called 911 and subsequently Mr. Peterson was admitted to Wellsford Community Hospital.

Even though the doctor recommends that Mr. Peterson be transferred to the subacute care unit of the hospital, Mr. and Mrs. Peterson
refuse to consider any discharge plan other than Mr. Peterson returning home. On August 14, Ms. McConnell meets with Nurse Shawna,
the hospital social worker, and Mr. and Mrs. Peterson to stipulate that
the Petersons need to allow the visiting nurse to resume services.
Ms. McConnell indicates that if the Petersons do not cooperate with
the plan, the adult protective services agency will consider whether
the situations warrant involuntary interventions.

What Nurse Roger Thinks

Although I'm not looking forward to dealing with this situation again,
at least I will have the support of Ms. McConnell and we will be working under the authority of adult protective services. Ms. McConnell
will meet me at the Petersons' house tomorrow and we'll visit together.
Ms. McConnell told me that Mr. Peterson thinks we are all "ganging
up on him" so I'll try to talk with him one-on-one and hope that he
begins to trust me. Mrs. Peterson seems to trust me so that is something I can build on. Ms. McConnell and I need to identify realistic
goals so we can keep this situation from escalating.

How Nurse Roger and Ms. McConnell Work Together

To: mcconnell@wcaps
From: nroger@wcvna
Subject: Peterson follow-up
Date: August 18

Thank you, Ms. McConnell, for visiting the Petersons with
me yesterday, as this is a challenging situation. I was pleased
to find that Mr. Peterson was using the oxygen, even though
it was not set at the correct dosage. As we discussed on the
phone, my immediate goal is to gain Mr. Peterson's trust, so
it was good that I had some time alone with him while you
stayed downstairs with Mrs. Peterson. Mr. Peterson seemed
a little less threatened this time, but I am concerned that if
we push for too much change he will close me out again.
Mr. Peterson needs to regain strength after being in bed for a
couple weeks and he did agree to have a physical therapist
visit to work with him, so I will arrange for that to begin later
this week.

To: nroger@wcvna
From: mcconnell@wcaps
Subject: Peterson follow-up
Date: August 20

Hello Nurse Roger,
Thanks for the update on the Petersons. If you can arrange
for a physical therapist, that will be a good start. I plan to
work with both Mr. and Mrs. Peterson to identify their needs
and offer resources and I hope that we can identify some
services that would be acceptable to the Petersons. Because
we both recognize that Mr. Peterson adamantly opposes the
use of outside services, I will approach the situation by
giving the Petersons choices. Also, I expect that I can identify
some resources that will not require them to pay out-of-
pocket. A home health aide would be covered by Medicare
as long as Mr. Peterson is getting skilled nursing or physical
therapy and the agency is certified as a provider by the
Centers for Medicare & Medicaid. I know your agency can
provide home health aides, but we also work with other
agencies for home care services. In this situation, a male aide
might be more acceptable and I know of an agency that
employs several male aides. What do you think about both
of us visiting to discuss this with the Petersons? Perhaps a
good strategy is for you to talk with Mr. Peterson and I will
talk with Mrs. Peterson. During my next visit, I will assess
Mrs. Peterson's needs using tools and suggestions from the
Family Caregiver Alliance. If we can arrange for a home
health aide to provide care for Mr. Peterson, then Mrs.
Peterson will have time for personal activities. In order for
her to continue her caregiving role, she needs respite and
help with coping. I'm hoping that I can get her to go to a
caregiver support group.

To: mcconnell@wcaps
From: nroger@wcvna
Subject: Peterson follow-up
Date: September 15

Hello Ms. McConnell,
I've visited the Petersons several times and am pleased that
the home health aide that you arranged continues to come

twice weekly. This has greatly improved Mr. Peterson's personal care and physical activity. Our physical therapist has directed the aide to follow through with an exercise program and Mr. Peterson is out of bed during much of the day. He is capable of going downstairs, but he has no motivation to leave his bedroom. Because we are at a standstill with any health-related goals, I will need to discharge this case in 2 weeks. The physical therapist will visit one more time, and after our skilled services are discontinued, the home health aide will not be covered by Medicare.

During my assessments, I identified some major indicators of depression and arranged for our mental health nurse practitioner to visit and she agreed that he would benefit from interventions for depression. As you are aware, he was diagnosed with dementia during his hospitalization, but the nurse practitioner is more concerned about depression, as his cognitive impairments are minimal at this point. Based on her assessment, the nurse practitioner is recommending a referral for mental health services. We cannot provide ongoing mental health services because he no longer meets the Medicare criterion for being homebound. Are you aware of mental health resources that might be appropriate in this situation?

To: nroger@wcvna
From: mcconnell@wcaps
Subject: Peterson follow-up
Date: September 18

Hello Nurse Roger,
Thank you for the update. Although I am disappointed that your agency will no longer be able to provide services, I understand your discharge plan and appreciate the assessment and recommendations of the mental health nurse practitioner. I have been working with Mrs. Peterson and, despite her attendance at several support group meetings, she is still struggling with issues surrounding being a caregiver, as she has indicated that she gets worn down due to his controlling behavior and lack of motivation toward

self-care. She continues to need respite from responsibilities and may also benefit from individual counseling. The Area Agency on Aging uses funds from the National Family Caregiver Support Program for Wellsford Catholic Social Services to provide caregiver counseling, and I will ask Mrs. Peterson if she'll agree to a referral. Also, our local adult day center has a contract with the county mental health agency to provide services for older adults with depression and I think this would be a good resource to address Mr. Peterson's issues and provide respite for Mrs. Peterson. Perhaps you could talk with Mr. Peterson about this as he seems to trust you now. Let's plan another joint visit to discuss these services with the Petersons before you discharge the case.

To: mcconnell@wcaps
From: nroger@wcvna
Subject: Peterson follow-up
Date: October 3

Dear Ms. McConnell,
I made my final visit to the Petersons yesterday and am pleased that Mr. Peterson agreed to attend the Wellsford Day Center program for 3 days a week starting next week. I mentioned that the weekly men's card club has been looking for new players and I told him this would be an opportunity to share his skills with others. He said, "I'll use it to show them some card tricks and prove that that incompetent doctor from the hospital doesn't know what he's talking about saying I have dementia." I think the program will help address his depression and motivate him to maintain self-care and manage his medical conditions. Also, as his dementia progresses, this will be a good resource for care, as I understand that the Wellsford Day Center program addresses the needs of people with dementia. Mrs. Peterson reported that she likes the counselor that you connected her with and also feels that she benefits from attending the support group. I understand that your agency will be following up with her and I would appreciate knowing what develops.

To: nroger@wcvna
From: mcconnell@wcaps
Subject: Peterson follow-up
Date: November 25

Dear Nurse Roger,
As requested, I am letting you know what has developed with
the Peterson case. I am pleased to report that Mrs. Peterson
continues with weekly visits to her counselor and monthly
support group meetings. She is coping better with her
caregiving situation and she appreciates the respite time while
Mr. Peterson attends day services three times a week. She has
resumed her volunteer activities with the Altar and Rosary
Society, which she gave up several months ago. The nurse at
the Wellsford Day Center reports that Mr. Peterson is less
depressed and his medical conditions are managed well.
Despite some noticeable cognitive impairments, he engages in
activities, including the men's card club. Surprisingly, he even
participates in the woodworking group and made a small
wooden trinket box. Our agency will be discharging the case
after I make a final visit next month.

KEY POINTS: WHAT NURSES NEED TO KNOW AND CAN DO

- Assess patterns of bruises to identify those that may be inflicted
  by others.
- Observe communication between older adults, spouses, friends,
  caregivers, and others.
- Arrange for caregivers and family members to have private
  conversations with health care professionals about concerns
  related to the situation.
- Be alert for signs of caregiver stress.
- Document assessment findings and discuss concerns and
  observations with other health care professionals.
- Initiate referrals for further assessment and appropriate services.
- Develop opportunities to work with professionals from other
  disciplines, such as social workers, mental health professionals,
  and rehabilitation therapists, to create a multidisciplinary team
  approach for addressing complex situations.

A NURSE IN ACTION CARING FOR A SELF-NEGLECTING OLDER ADULT

This chapter discusses the case of "Jane," a composite of various cases encountered by Georgia Anetzberger in her social work experiences in a rural county in northern Ohio. The case and accompanying material was published in *The Clinical Management of Elder Abuse* in 2005 and is currently used in gerontology courses to teach about multidisciplinary approaches to elder abuse. Each member of the multidisciplinary team, which included a nurse, physician, attorney, and social worker, described his or her discipline-specific approach to the situation during a team meeting led by Georgia Anetzberger. In addition, the chapter includes material developed by each team member describing professional perspectives on self-neglect. As with the case in Chapter 12, the nursing content is based on this author's clinical experiences. Note that as per physician orders, Nurse Anne visited Jane three times a week but this case presentation describes nursing actions and reflections only for intermittent visits. This approach provides an ongoing description as the case evolves. References and permissions are cited at the end of the chapter.

OVERVIEW: JANE

Outside, the wind is blowing off Lake Erie, threatening yet another blanket of snow on top of the five feet already accumulated in this rural county in northern Ohio. Jane looks out of the only window not hidden behind mounds of clutter, including books and papers from her days as a high school history teacher, furniture and appliances from flea market sales and her parents' estate, and piles of newspapers and clothing to sort and sell. Snow drifts submerge half of what used to be a barn near the house, now mostly fallen and rotting timber. The road is impassable. For some, the isolation imposed by the weather might be lonely and frightening, but Jane is not one of these people. She has nearly always managed on her own.

Jane is 78 years old and almost a lifelong resident of the county. An only child of farmers, she decided to become a teacher because "I was smarter than the other kids, and liked to boss people." She completed both her bachelor's and master's degrees by working various jobs when she attended college in neighboring counties. After graduation, she taught in an urban public school system, living in a small apartment nearby. Although never one to make friends willingly (some call her "aloof," others say "she thinks she's better than the rest of us"), Jane became attracted to a fellow teacher. The two women eventually decided to live together and bought a house on 30 acres of land in Jane's home county.

For nearly a quarter century, life for the two women had a certain routine. It was simple and pleasant, and it did not involve other people after Jane's parents died a few years into the couple's relationship. Daily tasks surrounded teaching and maintaining a garden, as well as several chickens and goats. The couple's main diversions were flea markets. And, of course, there were their cats, an ever growing number and assortment of strays that found their way to the women's property.

When her partner died suddenly and unexpectedly from complications following surgery, Jane became severely depressed, even further withdrawn, angry at the world, and bitter about her circumstances. Only the cats and home routine seemed to sustain her. Shortly after her partner's death, Jane retired with a pension for 30 years of service. The break from anyone associated with her job was immediate and complete.

If Jane remained sober, the pain of her partner's death was all-encompassing. Alcohol helped to make life bearable and eventually represented her "loyal old friend." During Jane's college days, she had frequented the gay bars in nearby cities, as was part of lesbian culture and identity during the 1950s. Everyone was very closeted then. Those in public service occupations, like Jane, had to be especially careful about employers discovering their sexual orientation because this could lead to loss of jobs, housing, and even freedom (jail was not out of the question). Jane left the bars behind when she met her partner; however, drinking remained something she did, perhaps not a lot, but certainly daily. Now she drinks a lot every day.

The snow continues to fall and the temperature drops. The only source of heat for the entire house is the living room fireplace, which Jane feeds with wood that she cut from fallen trees on her land. Despite the fire, the house is still cold and it hurts to lift the heavy logs. The furnace has not operated in 10 years and electricity is used for lights and cooking. Jane wears many layers of shirts, sweaters, and pants. Her feet are warmed by woolen socks and papers stuffed in extra-sized boots. She wears a thick woolen hat and lined leather work gloves. Jane has not changed her clothes for weeks—it is too cold, not necessary, and why bother, she believes.

The sparks dance from the fireplace. Mostly they land on surrounding stone. When a stray spark leaps onto a mound of clutter, Jane usually manages to crush it out before it causes any damage. Lately, she is missing more, because her eyesight is failing, or she is not getting there on time, because her arthritis is more disabling. Yesterday, sparks destroyed a chair and Jane burned her hands in the process of extinguishing the fire. The physician at the local urgent care center dressed the wounds, and told her that a visiting nurse would be coming to change the dressings. The charred chair remains where it was, a memorial to Jane's determination to manage on her own.

No outsider has entered the house in 20 years. Neighbors learned long ago to stay away and even though the house and land were viewed as "eyesores," few people are around to see them. Jane's only living relative is a distant cousin in Michigan, whose last contact resulted in an argument that made further contact unlikely. The number of cats has increased to about 30. Jane does not keep track of the count because some are inside cats and others are barn cats, and the barn cats come and go, often returning in the company of more.

Jane used to go to town monthly to buy groceries and other supplies but the trip will have to wait until better weather, even though little food remains. Driving used to be easier before Jane's eyesight worsened. Now it is hard to see details, and impossible to navigate at night. But what makes driving really hard is the prospect of getting lost. After a nearby intersection was closed, the route became unfamiliar, even confusing at times. Recently, it took a couple hours to make the usual 30-minute trip to town. Jane tries to remember if she had breakfast this morning, and cannot. "It doesn't really matter, I suppose," she reasons.

VISITING NURSE ANNE, FIRST VISIT TO JANE, FEBRUARY 12—INITIAL IMPRESSIONS AND ASSESSMENT

As the visiting nurse for this county, I had orders from the doctor at the Urgicare Center to visit three times a week for dressing changes. When I knocked at Jane's door for my initial visit, she yelled for me to come in. She was sitting on the couch, which was near the remains of the burnt chair. A fire was blazing in the fireplace, which had no screen in front of it. An ample supply of wood was next to the fireplace, with a stack of old newspaper next to it. She apologized for not getting up, saying, "I'm just too slow with my old Arthur bones." Jane was wearing a dirty terry cloth robe and frayed and worn out oversized slippers. I suspected that the slippers originally belonged to someone else. Her hair was matted and disheveled and I noted that her feet and ankles were swollen. Her eyes were bloodshot. A glass half-filled with a clear dark liquid sat on the table next to her, and when I did a "sniff test" I was sure it was some sort of hard liquor. Another "sniff test" confirmed the presence of old urine, presumably in the couch and floor. When I checked her blood pressure, I positioned myself to smell her breath, and sure enough, I detected an alcohol sweet aroma. Four cats checked me out from the other room, and I guessed that at least four more were around the house. When I first entered Jane's house, I was taken aback by the clutter, the bleak-looking environment, and the mix of odors from smoke, urine, and cats that permeated the stale air.

During the 10 years I had worked in this rural county, I had seen a variety of situations and met hundreds of people who had grown up in this area. Because Jane was like so many other lifelong residents of the county, I wasn't too concerned about her isolation. What I was concerned about, however, was the dearth of groceries and her seeming unawareness of the need to plan for getting more food and other supplies. Luckily, I had all the supplies that I needed for changing the burn dressings. I knew she wouldn't be able to drive until her hands healed and I wondered how she would get food for herself and the cats.

Jane told me she had plenty of food, but when I was in the kitchen washing my hands and she could not see me from the living room, I had sneaked a peek in her cupboards. The total supply of food in her house consisted of an almost-empty box of powdered milk, three boxes of macaroni and cheese, and not more than eight canned goods, mostly soups, corn, tuna fish, and corned beef hash. A couple bottles of apricot brandy were in the refrigerator, along with some rancid cheese and rotten lettuce. I estimated that the open bag of dry cat food wouldn't last for more than a couple days, considering that at least eight cats were living in Jane's house. I noted that the kitchen trash can contained three empty bourbon bottles, and I guessed that apricot brandy was Jane's "backup" drink. I suspected that Jane would be more concerned about the dwindling supply of apricot brandy and cat food than she would be about her own supply of food.

I wasn't sure if what I assessed as her "unawareness" arose from lack of insight, her long-term pattern of privacy, or her staunch spirit of self-sufficiency. I was sure she'd be upset if she knew I looked in her cupboards, so I needed to use the information about her food supply cautiously. Jane told me that the neighbor from a few miles away came at least weekly to see if she needed any groceries. When I inquired about the neighbor's name, she said, "She just goes by the name of 'Sally'." When I inquired about what day of the week Sally comes, she said, "Oh, I never know. It's whenever she happens by this neck of the woods." I observed that Jane did not have any calendars visible and the only clock I could see was in the kitchen. When I asked questions as my subtle way of assessing Jane's mental status, she was very vague or she answered with another question for me. For example, when I asked her if she knew what day of the week it was, she said, "What's the matter with you? Don't you know? Why do you have to ask me?" She was inventive in managing to dodge answers to many of my questions.

When I was changing the dressings on Jane's hands, I asked how she was managing to get things done, like getting washed, going to the bathroom, and preparing food. She said she was managing just fine, although she did acknowledge being a "little slow because of old Arthur" (i.e., her arthritis). She refused to show me how she walked or managed any of her other daily activities and she cut off my questions by saying, "Sally will come by if I need anything." She told me that Sally didn't have a phone so she couldn't give me any number for her. Sally's address was simply "the farmhouse up the road a bit." At one point during my visit, Jane stated, "You ask too many questions. It's too bad you need to keep coming back because you're a bit too nosey to suit me."

Nurse Anne's Thoughts After Her First Visit

I need a better assessment of Jane's mental status, but I sure don't know how I'll get it. I suspect she has some memory problems that she's trying desperately to cover up, but I could be wrong. I also suspect she was drinking apricot brandy right before my visit, but she's entitled to enjoy whatever she wants, since she's not diabetic as far as I know. Of course, she hasn't had any medical care for years, except what was done yesterday at the Urgicare Center, so maybe she does have some medical problems. I doubt that they did any blood tests. Her feet and ankles were swollen, but mine would be, too, if I sat down all day and the only thing I ate was canned food. I was afraid to suggest a homemaker or home-delivered meals, since she was adamant that Sally takes care of whatever she needs. I suspect that "Sally" exists only in Jane's mind, but I may never find that out, and certainly I won't get any further if Jane doesn't begin to trust me. I doubt that Jane is able to use that old-fashioned can opener because of the bandages on her hands and I considered offering to open a couple cans of food, but I'm sure she'd tell me that Sally would do that.

The referral from the Urgicare Center indicated that she is supposed to see a burn specialist for follow-up in a week. She insisted that she'll call the number on the paper and that Sally will take her, so I can't say much about that to her. I wonder if she can even use a telephone with those bandages. I think she called 911 when she couldn't put the fire out, so I know she called for help at least that one time.

I noticed a couple of fire hazards, but I'm not sure how I can approach her on that. There's no screen in front of the fireplace, and she keeps a stack of newspapers right near the open fireplace. I noted burn marks on the floor and I'm guessing that she's had spark fires. She doesn't have smoke detectors, but she told me that Sally offered to get one for her. I sure have a hard time fighting all of Sally's help! I don't think Jane moves much from the couch, so she's likely to notice if there is a fire—at least if she is awake and alert enough! On the other hand, her judgment and awareness seem impaired, so she's more likely to get burned and not be able to get help. I think I'll ask my supervisor if our agency can dip into our "Cookie Jar Fund" and buy her a screen for her fireplace. Of course, she'd have to be able to move it to put wood on the fire, so we would have to shop for the best kind for her. I've used that visiting nurse charity fund for other worthy causes and this would be a good way to resolve one safety hazard. I can call the fire department and ask them to come by with a smoke detector—they can tell Jane that this is their routine whenever they know about a fire. Maybe they will check around for other fire hazards and talk to her about some safety issues. I worry that Jane can't move very fast to get away from a fire. At least she keeps her phone nearby and can call 911. I almost tripped on the phone cord that stretches across the pathway between the living room and the kitchen. Maybe when I visit again, she'll let me rearrange the cord so it's not a fall hazard.

I need to develop a plan for getting more food in the house, because it will be a month before her hands are healed enough for the bandages to be removed and she certainly can't drive with her hands in this condition. Of course, I can't challenge the information about Sally too much, and I doubt that she cares much about whether or not she has food—I'm sure she cares a lot more about her supply of bourbon and apricot brandy and perhaps even about cat food. Maybe when she runs out of her "essentials," she'll let me arrange for grocery shopping.

NURSE ANNE'S THIRD VISIT, FEBRUARY 16—JANE'S CONTINUING ALTERNATE SENSE OF REALITY

This is the third time I've visited Jane, and she is sitting on the couch, looking pretty much the same as she did the last two times I visited. The odors from cats and urine are getting stronger. I can tell from the trash can in the kitchen that she had used the macaroni and cheese and another bottle of apricot brandy. Jane reports that Sally stopped by twice this week and brought her food, but there's no evidence of any new supplies. She reports that Sally will be taking her to the appointment with the burn specialist next week. She emphasizes that Sally has been a great help and she's glad she can count on her. After my last visit, Jane removed the bandages from the fingers on her right hand and today she refuses to let me put bandages on any of her fingers. I tell her that I need to put dressings on all her fingers and both hands because that's what the doctor ordered. When she sees the burn doctor on Tuesday, she can ask him about having some of the bandages off. She again assures me that Sally comes over to help with anything she needs and says, "You needn't mind my business about food—do I look like I'm starving?"

Nurse Anne's Thoughts After Her Third Visit

If anyone had been to see Jane since my last visit, I would see car tracks in the snow and the only ones I see are the ones from my car. I suspect that I've been the only visitor all week. I think Sally is a figment of Jane's imagination and she becomes "real" only when Jane needs to respond to my questions. I'm not sure how I can challenge this or get to the bottom of her reality. I suspect that Jane will have the dressings off when I come on Monday, because she can't manage the can opener with those bandages on. I again offered to arrange for home-delivered meals, but she told me that Sally was bringing food later today. I need to appreciate that Jane leaves the door unlocked and lets me come in and I don't want to threaten the delicate relationship I have with her by pushing for homemaker services or any other outside help. No matter what questions I ask, her answers are vague. She's quite clever in her responses; I can tell she's an educated woman. Based on my assessment during these three visits, I'm sure that Jane has some memory problems, but maybe she has some medical conditions that are causing some cognitive impairment—or maybe the apricot brandy is a contributing factor. Whatever is going on, I wish I could get her assessed because I hate to overlook anything that's treatable.

Someone as private and independent as Jane would do best if she can stay in her own home, but if her judgment is impaired, she would be at risk staying there alone. I feel a responsibility to make sure that any medical conditions are identified so Jane can at least decide if she wants to have treatments. Of course, alcohol is likely to be a contributing factor, and she is not likely to agree to stop drinking. I think her apricot brandy is more of a "real" friend than Sally is. Perhaps it's best to just respect her privacy and let her live her life with her alcohol and her cats. It does bother me, though, that I might be overlooking something treatable. If I ignore this situation, it's certain to deteriorate and she's sure to end up back at the Urgicare Center. Even worse, she might have a serious fire or another life-threatening problem and not even be able to call for help.

I think I'll contact the burn doctor she's seeing on Tuesday and find out if he will suggest that she goes to Dr. J. M. because he has been so good with other patients who have needed a good assessment. If I can get Jane to see Dr. J. M., at least he would check for medical problems and assess her mental status so we have some idea about her cognitive functioning. If Jane had a medical problem that could be easily addressed, I could talk with her about taking care of the medical issues as a way of maintaining her independence and staying in her own home. Maybe if I am friendlier with her cats, she'll trust me and open up a little more to me.

I noticed that there's a smoke detector in the living room and I was pleased that the fire department had followed through with this. This might be backfiring, though, because when I told Jane I was glad to see the smoke detector, she said, "See, I told you Sally would be coming by and she brought the smoke detector just like I told you she would." Now it will be even more difficult to challenge Sally's existence because I don't want to let her know that I asked the fire department to install the smoke detector. Besides, if I challenge anything Jane tells me about Sally, it will ruin the fragile relationship I've been able to develop. When I told her I was bringing a fireplace screen that I had been storing in my basement, she said, "Well, I guess I'll have two of them then, because Sally's bringing one next week. But, if you want to get rid of some trash in your basement, that's OK with me."

NURSE ANNE'S FIFTH VISIT, FEBRUARY 20—IMPLEMENTING NEW COMMUNICATIONS STRATEGIES; SOME PROGRESS OCCURRING

As usual, Jane is sitting on the couch, wearing the same clothing she had on when I first visited. I brought the fireplace screen after I removed all the labels and added a little dust so it looked a little used. I place it in front of the burning fire and I ask Jane if I can move the stack of papers off to the side. She tells me that the screen that Sally is getting her will be a lot nicer, and adds, "I'll keep your basement trash for now if it makes you happy." I tell her that it will make me very happy. She has removed the bandages from all her fingers since my last visit and I ask how her appointment with the burn specialist was yesterday. She says that Sally had car trouble, so she rescheduled the appointment for next week. I'm relieved that her burns are healing despite the fact that she takes the dressing off.

I make a conscious effort to improve my relationship with Jane by asking about the names of her cats and she rattles off eight names. Despite my allergies, I extend my hands to the friendliest of the cats and I show interest in the one who comes to rub against me. I engage Jane in extended conversation about the cats, and I work my way up to asking about whether she'll be needing food for the cats. When I checked the supply of cat food, I noted that it was dangerously low. My nose tells me that the kitty litter is totally saturated and useless. She relies on her usual Sally response, and I gather up enough courage to say, "If Sally is having car problems, she might not be reliable enough— I'm sure you want to be certain that you have enough food for all these four-legged friends of yours." My strategy isn't entirely successful, but she admits, "If you come back before Sally gets here again, I guess you can bring some cat food." When I suggest that the county senior program would send someone to do the grocery shopping, she adamantly says, "You can bring some cat food if you've got some stored in your basement, but don't be sending no do-gooder to help me when I don't need any help. Sally's car is going to be fixed tomorrow. I told you to keep out of my business."

Nurse Anne's Thoughts After Her Fifth Visit

I'm disappointed that Jane didn't go to the burn doctor because his office nurse said they'd try to get Jane to see Dr. J. M. If Jane doesn't keep her appointment with the burn doctor and she's not compliant about keeping the dressing on, then she won't qualify for skilled nursing visits from my agency any longer. At least she certainly meets the "homebound" requirement for Medicare. I suspect she'll begin to drive if there's no other way to get cat food and alcohol, and I wonder if she's safe driving. The nearest store is 11 miles away and some of the roads are still snow covered. Even if I got her some groceries and cat food, she'll want bourbon and brandy and homemakers from the county might not get that for her. My supervisor approved of buying the fireplace screen from our Cookie Jar fund, but I doubt she'll approve of more expenditures and I'm surely not going to ask about buying alcohol for Jane. I wish I could get a better assessment of Jane's mental status. As I talk with her, I note a lot of evidence about memory problems and impaired judgment. The only evidence of medical problems is that her feet and ankles are always swollen but she appears to be very underweight and I am concerned about her nutritional status. I also see evidence of urinary incontinence and I wonder if she has a urinary tract infection.

At least I've made some progress with the safety issues, but I still don't know if she can make any phone calls, except for 911. I finally got her permission to move the phone cord from the pathway, but there's still a lot of extension cords across the floor and they look unsafe. I'd like to look at the bedroom and bathroom to check for hazards but she's already accused me of being too nosey. If I push her too far, I'm sure she'll have the door locked the next time I come. I can see that she'll never accept any home-delivered meals or homemaker service for grocery shopping. Besides, if I make a referral to the county senior assistance program, the homemaker would want to clean the kitchen and do some laundry and that would be the end of any services as far as Jane is concerned.

NURSE ANNE'S LAST VISIT, FEBRUARY 24—FINAL IMPRESSIONS AND ASSESSMENT

As soon as I pull into the driveway at Jane's house, I notice that her car has been cleared off and is now parked in a different place. Jane is sitting on her couch as usual and calls for me to come in. She looks pretty much the same except there are no bandages on her hands. She tells me she won't be needing me again because her hands are all better. I examine her hands and assess that the burns are 80% healed, but there are some deep scabs and reddened areas. She does not have full range of motion for her fingers and it looks like some of the burn wounds are on the verge of infection. I am also concerned that she could get contractures where the scar tissue is forming. As usual, she insists that she doesn't need any help with anything. I check the cupboards when I am in the kitchen and I find four bottles of bourbon and four bottles of apricot brandy, a supply of cat food, and several cans of soup. Jane tells me that Sally stopped by and brought the groceries. She also says Sally will be taking her to the doctor appointment tomorrow, and there's no need for me to come back. Jane is going to keep the door locked from now on because she's seen a suspicious trail of footprints between her car and her front door. She emphasizes that she's not going to let anyone in, "including Miss Snoopy Nurse, even though you're a nice person."

Nurse Anne's Thoughts After Her Last Visit

I guess Jane is pretty self-sufficient. Even if she'd let me back in, Medicare wouldn't pay for the visit because she's not compliant with the treatment. She's got what she needs to survive. I've addressed some of the safety concerns, but I sure do wonder about her mental status, especially her ability to make safe decisions. I also worry about her driving and I hope she's safe enough on the roads. I assessed that Jane has some cognitive impairments, and I suspect that there's at least one medical intervention that could be initiated to improve her functioning, but I don't think she'd cooperate with any treatment—especially if it involved giving up her brandy. But, on the other hand, she should have the benefit of an assessment, so a professional can talk to her about her choices. Maybe if she understands that giving up alcohol— or at least cutting down on how much she drinks—and getting treatment for any medical conditions could be the key to maintaining her independence in her own home, then she'd choose to cooperate. I know that independence and staying in her own home are extremely important to her. I'll discuss this situation with my supervisor because I'm not comfortable with just closing this case.

NURSE ANNE'S ACTION: REVIEW WITH SUPERVISOR SHEILA, FEBRUARY 27

Supervisor Sheila's Thoughts and Recommendation Including Identification of Associated Ethical Dilemmas Associated With This Case

Nurse Anne had a lot of barriers to deal with in establishing a relationship with Jane, who for so many years led a reclusive lifestyle. If she hadn't used some good communication techniques, she would never have been able to visit five times. She did not challenge Jane's statements about Sally, even though she had good reason to believe that Sally exists only in Jane's imagination. Also, Nurse Anne was friendly toward Jane's cats and used them as a topic of conversations so Jane would accept her a little more. Nurse Anne was astute in her observations and she informally assessed Jane's mental status as best she could. She also identified some major safety issues and found creative ways of addressing fire hazards and fall risks. Even though sneaking a look in Jane's cupboards might seem like a violation of privacy, it was important to find out if Jane had enough food for survival.

Ethical dilemmas that Nurse Anne dealt with included issues of freedom over safety and the right to personal choices, even when risks are involved. By resolving major safety issues in Jane's house, Nurse Anne reduced the risk and respected Jane's choice of living arrangements. She was also concerned about Jane's driving and potential risk to the safety of others, but she wasn't able to address this. Nurse Anne's other ethical dilemma was related to her professional responsibility to identify health problems that can be treated, while at the same time respecting Jane's right to refuse treatment. She had reason to believe that Jane had some treatable conditions and that Jane's health, functioning, and ability to remain independent would improve if these conditions were addressed. At a minimum, Jane should have the opportunity to make an informed decision about the potential outcomes of her choices. Nurse Anne was clever—but unsuccessful—in her attempt to arrange a referral for assessment. Because there are several loose ends involving ethical dilemmas, Nurse Anne can present this case at the next meeting of the County Elders-at-Risk Consultation Team. I've been participating in those meetings for several years and it's always reassuring to have feedback from the other members.

NURSE ANNE'S ACTION: PRESENTATION OF CASE FOR CONSULTATION AT COUNTY ELDERS-AT-RISK CONSULTATION TEAM, MARCH 14

The County Elders-at-Risk Consultation Team meets monthly to review cases presented by participating agencies. Supervisor Sheila has arranged for Nurse Anne to present her case for consultation.

Nurse Anne, After Summarizing the Case

"My biggest concern is that Jane gets a good geriatric assessment because she may have some unidentified medical conditions that could be managed to improve her functioning. I'm not sure I have enough evidence to make a report to adult protective services. There are a lot of people out there who are reclusive and perhaps living at some risk, but they're entitled to live the way they want."

Social Worker Carol, Representing County Adult Protective Services, Discussing the Role of Adult Protective Services and Advising Nurse Anne to Make a Report

"I think a report is warranted because you've entered the home in a situation that has been isolated and hidden for a long time. You identified characteristics of self-neglect and significant risks of fire and further injury. Jane doesn't realize the risks in her situation, nor does she appreciate that these risks are increasing. I understand that people don't like turning someone in to the government, which may come with a heavy hand and say, 'You can't live like this. You need to start changing things.' That's an unfortunate misrepresentation of what will happen, because the adult protective services social worker will be committed to respecting Jane's right to refuse services as long as she understands her risk and wants to stay. Because Jane has been so isolated, it may be that no one has made any offer to help. With her history and personality, it will take a concerted effort to melt down her resistance—it likely will be quite a while before Jane accepts help. In adult protective services, we begin as a neutral party. We try to convey that we neither believe nor disbelieve the report. We take it as a statement of concern. I think of adult protective services as an alarm clock that goes off in people's lives, alerting them that there are sufficient concerns that the government has become involved."

"Jane's lack of insight or motivation may be due to depression, and alcohol may be the only way she knows to cope with grief. Projecting a 'best-case scenario' for this situation, if an adult protective services worker could gain entry into Jane's private world, the social worker would try to establish a trusting relationship so Jane would open up about her life. The social worker would be assisted by the department's behavioral health nurse, who would develop a beginning understanding of Jane's profound grief at the loss of her partner. The social worker and behavioral health nurse would discuss with Jane the critical importance of having a thorough examination to identify causes of her increasing forgetfulness and confusion. Jane would agree to an assessment and her underlying issues would be addressed."

Attorney Maria, County Legal Aid Services, Describing Legal Implications

"If you referred Jane to adult protective services, an investigation would be triggered and it is likely that Jane would be found to be a self-neglecting older adult in need of services, according to our state law. It also is likely that Jane would refuse to consent to voluntary protective services if that would impinge on her privacy and freedom to live her life as she sees fit. An attorney would vigorously defend Jane's right to live as she chooses. As an advisor, the attorney may well attempt to counsel Jane to cooperate voluntarily with any recommended protective services. The advisor might point out that such cooperation could enhance her ability to continue to live safely in her home and to retain control over her life."

"Also, the attorney is obligated to advise Jane about the dangers and legal ramifications of driving while impaired. If the attorney thinks that Jane's driving poses a real and immediate risk of causing serious harm to others, the attorney has a duty to report such a belief to law enforcement authorities. Such a report would not trigger actions such as confiscation of her car, but it might bring yet another persuasive authority into her situation."

Doctor John, Geriatric Assessment Program, Describing the Role of Physicians, Commenting on Nurse Anne's Work, and Recommending a Referral

"It would seem that Jane needs to undergo some kind of medical assessment. I agree with what Social Worker Carol said about someone from adult protective services establishing a relationship with her and getting her to agree to an assessment. Certainly, she may have conditions that, if treated, would dramatically reduce her risks. If I could see her at our geriatric assessment clinic, I would focus on Jane's ability to live independently in her current home, address her medical concerns so that she feels better, and eventually I would help her develop some insight about her isolation and its effects. If adult protective services could gain Jane's cooperation for a medical evaluation, key tasks for me as her physician will include the establishment of a working relationship, diagnosis of possible medical issues, and addressing any questions about her decision-making capacity."

"As a physician I am responsible for evaluating and managing medical conditions that may be increasing a patient's vulnerability. Self-neglect strongly tests the balance between autonomy and beneficence and therefore presents conflicting ethical duties for health care professionals. Developing a physician–patient relationship involves learning what Jane's values, decisions, and priorities are and respecting them. It is then important to see if we can establish mutual goals. I would clarify my role and offer advice and recommendations, recognizing that these may clash with Jane's priorities. A good starting point is to focus on the mutual goal of optimizing her independence. If I can establish rapport with Jane, she might be willing to discuss some of the issues and concerns with me and the other members of our team at the clinic. Any approach is likely to be an uphill battle, but an attitude that respects Jane's intelligence is more likely to be successful than one that is condescending or authoritative."

"Jane's assessment should begin with her life history, in order to establish rapport and learn about her background and living situation. This process would provide assessment information about her memory, insight, and cognitive function. Assessment of her functional status will be more important than specific diagnoses in establishing her decision-making capacity, so I would arrange for an occupational therapy evaluation and include other professionals as warranted. If Jane is insightful and aware of her current situation and is making reasoned choices that are consistent with choices she has made throughout her life, we should respect her decisions, even though they may be unwise. I would reinforce my willingness to work with Jane to meet her goals and describe how each intervention would be directed toward helping Jane to maintain her optimal independence. It is also important to recognize the limits of what we can provide and to acknowledge and respect her intelligence. Presenting oneself as an all-knowing expert would be especially unsuccessful here."

"Nurse Anne, you've successfully gained entrance into Jane's life for five visits, and that's to your credit. At this point, though, I would recommend a referral to the county adult protective services and perhaps they can build on your efforts and gain enough trust that Jane would eventually agree to an assessment."

Social Worker Carol, Reflecting on Probable Scenarios

"If you reported the case, I would be the one making the initial visit and even if Jane doesn't accept any recommendations now, at least she will recognize me if we get another report and I visit again. It's pretty predictable that some crisis will occur and we'll hear about Jane from the sheriff or a concerned neighbor—as you know, we usually do. Out here in this county, situations like this don't resolve by themselves and someone is bound to become involved again. Perhaps we'll even be able to call upon you as a visiting nurse to help us with this."

KEY POINTS: WHAT NURSES NEED TO KNOW AND CAN DO

■ Nurses can be resourceful in obtaining as much assessment information as possible so they can consider risks in relation to the personal characteristics of the older adult.

■ Nurses can identify creative ways of addressing risks while respecting the older adult's autonomy.

■ Nurses can seek guidance from other professionals to address their concerns about older adults in at-risk situations.

REFERENCES

Material in this chapter has been adapted from the following citations, used with permission from Taylor and Francis.

Jane: Overview
Anetzberger, G. J. (2005). Elder abuse: Case studies for clinical management. In G. J. Anetzberger (Ed.), *The clinical management of elder abuse* (pp. 43–53). New York, NY: Haworth Press.

Social Worker Carol
Dayton, C. (2005). Elder abuse: The social worker's perspective. In G. J. Anetzberger (Ed.), *The clinical management of elder abuse* (pp. 135–155). New York, NY: Haworth Press.

Doctor John
McGreevey, J. F. (2005). Elder abuse: The physician's perspective. In G. J. Anetzberger (Ed.), *The clinical management of elder abuse* (pp. 83–103). New York, NY: Haworth Press.

Nurse Anne
Miller, C. A. (2005). Elder abuse: The nurse's perspective. In G. J. Anetzberger (Ed.), *The clinical management of elder abuse* (pp. 105–133). New York, NY: Haworth Press.

Attorney Maria
Schimer, M. (2005). Elder abuse: The attorney's perspective. In G. J. Anetzberger (Ed.), *The clinical management of elder abuse* (pp. 43–53). New York, NY: Haworth Press.

A NURSE AS A MEMBER OF A MULTIDISCIPLINARY TEAM PREVENTING ELDER ABUSE

Nursing involvement to prevent elder abuse can be viewed as a health promotion intervention in that it addresses conditions that increase the risk of an unhealthy situation from deteriorating into abuse. Although the roles of nurses in addressing risks have been discussed throughout this book, this chapter focuses on keeping one step ahead of abuse by addressing conditions that have a high probability of developing into an abusive situation. These risks can be identified in both the older adult and the potential perpetrator by using the Benjamin Rose Institute on Aging's (BRIA) Risk of Abuse Tool to identify vulnerabilities associated with increased risk. Using information based on this tool, professionals can implement interventions in a timely manner with the intent of preventing abuse from occurring. The case example in this chapter describes ways in which a nurse and other members of a multidisciplinary team use the tool to identify and address risks to prevent a potentially abusive situation from escalating. For nurses, the case illustrates the importance of using nursing interventions not only to address usual health-related goals but also to achieve the additional goal of preventing elder abuse. In addition, it illustrates how a nurse functions within a multidisciplinary team to address multifaceted needs of both the older adult and the caregiver.

Content of this chapter was developed by the BRIA in Cleveland, Ohio, for this book. In addition to engaging in applied research and public policy advocacy, BRIA provides a wide range of home and community-based services and programs, including home health care and affordable, independent housing geared toward promoting the safety, health, and independent functioning of older adults in their homes (BRIA, n.d.). The BRIA's Risk of Abuse Tool and the Recognizing Abuse Tool described in Chapter 7 are examples of research-based tools that this agency developed for clinical practice. The fictitious case in this chapter illustrates how a multidisciplinary team, including a nurse, uses the Risk of Abuse Tool to develop interventions that are directed toward preventing abuse from occurring.

The chapter first provides an overview of the Risk of Abuse Tool and then describes the application of this tool in a community-based clinical setting. The information is applicable to nurses in all settings because it illustrates how usual nursing interventions can be effective in reducing risks and preventing the occurrence of elder abuse. Nurses do not always know if their interventions are successful in preventing abuse from occurring in the long term; however, they can experience satisfaction from knowing that their interventions addressed immediate risks. In addition, interventions directed toward the prevention of abuse are likely to improve health and functioning of the older adult, which are goals by themselves.

OVERVIEW OF THE RISK OF ABUSE TOOL

The Risk of Abuse Tool was developed to fill the need for a screening tool that focuses on prevention of abuse, rather than on indicators of actual or suspected abuse. The development of the tool was based on an earlier training that was empirically tested and used with adult protective service workers in Ohio (Anetzberger, 2006; Bass, Anetzberger, Ejaz, & Nagpaul, 2001; Ejaz, Bass, Anetzberger, & Nagpaul, 2001). In 2014, the final tool and a related online training program were released for use by care managers participating in a demonstration program to coordinate care for dually eligible Medicare and Medicaid populations in 29 of Ohio's 88 counties (Ejaz, Bukach, Conway, & Anetzberger, 2014). As of August 2015, 453 care managers enrolled in the training (Anetzberger & Ejaz, 2016). The tool defines *abuse* broadly to include various types, including physical, sexual, and emotional abuse; neglect; and exploitation. A unique characteristic of this tool is its focus on vulnerabilities of a "possible" victim and/or a possible perpetrator that make them susceptible to abusive situations. Thus, the tool is used before actual abuse has occurred; therefore, neither party should be labeled as a victim or an abuser. Another important characteristic is that the tool pertains to risks in both the possible victim and the possible perpetrator, rather than to those related only to the older adult.

The Risk of Abuse Tool has five general sections, each representing a category of risk: (a) past abuse, neglect, exploitation, or criminal offenses; (b) relationship problems; (c) physical, emotional, or mental health-related problems; (d) caregiving and support; and (e) environmental and household characteristics. Although these categories are distinct, questions are often interrelated. For example, the section on relationship problems is likely to be related to the section on emotional or mental health-related issues. Another consideration is that because additional risk factors may be present, professionals are encouraged to supplement the questions with information based on their clinical judgment. Items on the tool can be used in any of the following ways: (a) to develop questions for clients/patients, (b) to document observations about the presence of a risk factor, or (c) to elicit information from others (e.g., friends, professionals, family). Professionals can also use the tool in a variety of situations, such as when the older adult has dementia or when the professional has no prior knowledge of or contact with a possible perpetrator. Questions are applicable to both the possible victim and the possible perpetrator unless the box in one column is blacked out. The intent of this tool is to identify risks of abuse; however, if indicators of actual or suspected abuse are identified, the professional should use the Recognizing Abuse Tool (described in Chapter 7) and follow appropriate reporting protocols.

The case of Elsa illustrates how professionals use this tool to identify and address risks for abuse. As the case unfolds, risks of abuse are shown in italics to correspond with questions that are checked off in the Risk of Abuse Tool in Figure 14.1.

CASE OVERVIEW: ELSA

More than 50 years ago, Elsa, a teenager, and her older husband, Joseph, emigrated from their homeland, which was plagued by war, seeking the promise of a fresh start in the United States. They had witnessed too much violence in their town and lost everything they had, except a few treasured possessions and each other. Despite their initial fear as they arrived in a strange country, they settled in Cleveland, Ohio, and Joseph found work in a manufacturing plant. Joseph was an authoritarian figure who took great pride in his role as a man taking responsibility for providing well for his family. Elsa was obedient and loyal,

FIGURE 14.1   Risk of Abuse Tool as applied to Elsa.

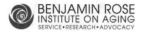
BENJAMIN ROSE
INSTITUTE ON AGING
SERVICE•RESEARCH•ADVOCACY

RISK OF ABUSE TOOL©

Name of Client:____*Elsa*_____   Case Number: :__*1003762*_____

The Risk of Abuse Tool identifies factors in the literature commonly associated with being at risk for abuse in the future. It is designed as a resource to help you gather information about an individual's risk for abuse. It includes both possible victim and possible perpetrator characteristics. Please remember that this tool can be used without having any knowledge about the perpetrator.

A question intended for both possible victim and possible perpetrator is identified by non-shaded columns next to the corresponding screening question. A question intended for a possible victim only is shaded in the column referring to the possible perpetrator and vice-versa. If a risk factor is present, indicate whether it is likely to occur in the possible victim, possible perpetrator, or both, by checking the appropriate box(es). If you believe an individual needs services, please contact the Aging and Disability Resource Network for advice. If you believe or suspect that the individual is experiencing abuse, please switch to using the Recognizing Abuse Tool, and follow the associated reporting protocol.

RISK FACTOR SCREENING QUESTIONS	Possible Victim (check)	Possible Perpetrator (check)
Past Abuse, Neglect, Exploitation, or Criminal Offenses		
Has the person experienced or witnessed abuse or other violence or criminal offenses? *Mark got a DUI*		✓
Has the person perpetrated abuse, criminal offenses or other violence toward another person/animal?		
Relationship Problems		
Is there a belief in strict gender roles? *Family's culture supports belief in strict gender roles*	✓	✓
Does the person have a history of coercing, manipulating, or asserting dominance, power or control over another individual? *Mark dominates his mother*		✓
Is the person extremely jealous or possessive of his/her spouse/significant other?		
Does one person have unrealistic expectations of the other?		
Is the possible victim planning to leave/has recently left an abusive relationship?		■
Physical, Emotional, or Mental Health-Related Problems		
Has the person suffered from a traumatic event (e.g. war or a natural disaster)? *Elsa fled from war*	✓	
Does the person lack understanding of the possible victim's medical condition? *Both lack knowledge of Elsa's condition*	✓	✓
Does the person have behavioral problems or issues with relationships, blaming others, or hostility?		
Does the person have a cognitive impairment or mental or emotional disorder? *Mark is depressed*	✓	
Does the person have an intellectual disability?		
Does the person have a physical impairment? *Because of her surgery, Elsa is functionally limited for now*	✓	
Does the person have problems with alcohol, drugs, or medications? *Mark struggles with alcoholism*		✓
Does the possible perpetrator have a history of work-related problems? *Mark's been fired many times*	■	✓
Does the possible victim lack a consistent primary care physician?		■
Caregiving and Support		
Does the person lack social support or is socially isolated? *Both have few friends*	✓	✓
Does the possible perpetrator have difficulty/reluctance with caregiving tasks for the possible victim? *Mark seems unwilling and has never been a caregiver before* ←	■	✓
Does the possible perpetrator have stress or inexperience related to care giving?		✓
Does the person have low socioeconomic status (e.g. poverty, financial dependency, low education)? *Mark is financially dependent on Elsa because he is out of work*		✓
Cultural, Environmental, or Household Characteristics		
Is violence justified or accepted in the person's culture or community?		
Do the possible victim and perpetrator share a household?	✓	✓
Does the possible perpetrator have access to a weapon, such as a gun?	■	
Does the house have hazardous environmental conditions (e.g. hoarding, rodents)? *Elsa is a hoarder*	✓	✓
Is the possible victim's neighborhood unsafe or high in crime?		

Used with permission from Ejaz et al. (2014).

and always had dinner ready on the table when her husband returned from work. She knew everything that a traditional wife should, including how to get a stain out of any fabric, and the trick to making a pair of good work boots last a few more months. After they gave birth to a baby, Mark, they bought a small house close to Joseph's work. The family lived modestly and joined a local church attended by other people from their homeland; they soon had a small community with which they identified. Like other newly arrived immigrants, they scrimped and saved to make ends meet, but Elsa went even further; she could not bear to part with anything. Even if an item had no use at all, she was compelled to save it because she might be able to reuse it. *She saved all these items in old cardboard boxes, stacked them up, and covered them (*hoarding). Over time, these boxes began taking up space all around the house.*

As Mark grew up and began attending school, Joseph made sure that his son learned the language, culture, and tradition of his heritage. Mark, on the other hand, wanted to conform to an American lifestyle and was resentful of his traditional upbringing. He hated the fact that his parents spoke poor English and had heavy accents. He constantly had to help them complete paperwork in English and talk on the phone because others could not understand them. When Mark was a teenager, his father fell seriously ill and passed away. After his father's death, Mark felt that he could finally live the American dream and break away from some of his family's traditionally held values. His mother, on the other hand, had to deal with many new responsibilities. Since Joseph's Social Security checks were not enough to make ends meet, Elsa began working as a seamstress in a garment factory within walking distance.

During this period, Mark lost interest in his education. He was out at all hours of the night, rarely checking in with his mother. At age 18, Mark viewed his legal independence as an escape and started working at a construction company. He moved across town, as far away from his childhood house as he could, and did not go back home unless his mother begged him to come for a delicious meal she made especially for him. During this time, *Mark began to drink (*problems with alcoholism).* He often came to work late and with a bad attitude; eventually, he was fired. From then on, Mark lost numerous jobs, always living paycheck to paycheck (**history of work-related problems*). By the time he was in his 50s, he was in a great deal of debt *and he became depressed (*mental health-related problems).* One day he was arrested for driving under the influence (DUI) of alcohol. After his release from jail, he moved in with his mother (*victim and perpetrator share a household*). As Elsa's friends moved away and different ethnic groups moved into the neighborhood, both Elsa and Mark became *very lonely (*socially isolated).* Elsa stopped attending church after Mark moved in with her and told her he no longer believed in the same God as she did. He frequently *made derogatory remarks about her friends at church* and *distanced himself from them (*relationship problems).*

Elsa felt responsible for providing housing for her son and she appreciated that he at least did the heavy work around the house when she asked for help. Elsa cooked meals for both of them, but neither she nor Mark did much housekeeping. Elsa and Mark *ignored the piles of clutter that were accumulating (*hoarding)* and both seemed content to have a narrow pathway between the bedrooms and bathrooms. Elsa continued to work past retirement age because her Social Security income was minimal and Mark had no source of income. By the time Elsa was in her 70s, she was in constant pain from arthritis and was taking medications for hypertension and type 2 diabetes. She *had difficulty walking (*physical impairment)* and always felt exhausted. Several years ago, she began using a glucometer to check her blood sugar, but she stopped doing that months ago after the glucometer broke. Elsa suspected that her A1C was higher than it should be, but she had no motivation to follow a healthy diet.

When Elsa was returning from work one day, she slipped and fell as she was going up the steps into the house. She was taken to the emergency department, where she was diagnosed with osteoporosis, hypertension, uncontrolled diabetes, and a fractured hip. During her admission for hip surgery, Mark visited daily.

NURSE RAYMOND, ELSA'S CASE MANAGER, CLEVELAND HOSPITAL, ADDRESSING CONCERNS ABOUT ELSA'S DISCHARGE PLAN

Elsa's postsurgical course was uneventful; however, her A1C on admission was 8.6 and her blood pressure was 186/98. Nurse Raymond observed that Elsa frequently ate cookies and chocolate candy that Mark brought. He also noted Mark's breath smelled like alcohol and his eyes were bloodshot. Mark never asked questions about his mother's care and he seemed to avoid any contact with Nurse Raymond. When Nurse Raymond talked with Elsa about being transferred to a rehabilitation unit in the hospital, Elsa insisted on being discharged to home where Mark could care for her. Despite Nurse Raymond's best effort, he was unable to convince Elsa to go to a rehabilitation unit, but she did agree to a referral for home health care services. Prior to discharge, Nurse Raymond reviewed wound care with Elsa and the registered dietician met with Elsa for diabetic diet instructions. Nurse Raymond had asked Mark to be present for these instructions, but Mark did not come to the hospital until Elsa had already signed all discharge papers and had all her belongings packed. When he came to accompany her home, Elsa insisted that they needed to leave right away because Mark's friend was waiting in the car to take them home. Elsa was referred to the BRIA because the agency provides a variety of community-based services including home health care, social services, mental health services, and low-income housing for seniors. Nurse Cathy was assigned to make the initial visit to assess the situation and recommend interventions.

NURSE CATHY, COMMUNITY-BASED NURSE, PERFORMING INITIAL ASSESSMENT, RECOGNIZING RISKS, AND IMPLEMENTING INTERVENTIONS

When Nurse Cathy called to schedule an initial home visit, Mark answered the phone and said the services were not necessary; however, Nurse Cathy said she needed to talk with Elsa, who then agreed to the visit. When Nurse Cathy arrived at the house, she noted that the entry was unsafe because there was no railing on the side of the stairs. As part of her assessment, Nurse Cathy requested to see the house in order to identify risks to safety. She noted that there was no raised toilet seat or shower chair in the bathroom, despite the recommendation that was noted on the discharge summary. Elsa said she would be happy to have these installed, but Mark did not think they were worth what it would cost. Nurse Cathy also noted *a maze of old newspapers, magazines, and dirty cardboard boxes all around the house (*hoarding)*, leaving only narrow pathways for walking. Prior to discharge, Elsa had used a walker, but she was unable to use one at home because of the cluttered walkways. Nurse Cathy expressed concerns about Elsa falling again and explained the importance of clearing the clutter and cleaning the house to create safe walkways.

Nurse Cathy suggested that a home health aide come three times a week to help Elsa with bathing and dressing. In order to personalize the plan of care, Nurse Cathy sought input from Elsa about her preferences for days and times that would work best for her to have someone in the house. She also recommended physical therapist visits to help Elsa gain strength with mobility. Nurse Cathy spoke to Mark about helping his mother with her activities of daily living and housework when home care staff was not there. Nurse Cathy discussed additional nursing goals related to diabetes management and wound care, including infection prevention related to the incision in her hip. When Nurse Cathy referred to Mark as the primary family caregiver for his mother, she recognized that both Mark and Elsa were feeling overwhelmed. They appeared *confused by all the medical issues and how long it would take Elsa to recover (*both lacked understanding of the possible victim's medical condition)*. Mark appeared visibly upset and *expressed* *his reluctance about taking on the caregiving role (*reluctance with caregiving tasks for the possible victim).* Cathy assured him that the BRIA home health care team would be there to provide ongoing assistance and help, and address any concerns he had. She felt that she was able to dispel some of his distress.

NURSE CATHY'S FOLLOW-UP VISIT, IDENTIFYING ADDITIONAL RISKS AND FACILITATING A TEAM APPROACH

During the follow-up home visit, Nurse Cathy noticed the new hand rail outside the house. When she went inside the house, she requested to see whether the raised toilet seat and hand rails had been installed and saw that they were. She thanked Mark for his role in helping to install these. However, she was taken aback by Mark's response. He began to hyperventilate, explaining that he did not have a life anymore and felt homebound due to his mother's condition (*having stress or inexperience related to caregiving*). He also stressed that it was his mother's duty to get well so she could resume all the household responsibilities; *she was, after all, the only woman in the house (*belief in strict gender roles).* Elsa, too, was tearful and explained that she felt helpless, and kept repeating that she was not being a good mother at this time. *She felt that because Mark was a man, he shouldn't have to do any of the housework while she was still alive (*belief in strict gender roles).* When Cathy asked Mark about his availability to help during the day, she realized that *he was unemployed (*financial dependency)* and frustrated by his situation. She also suspected that he *had been drinking (*alcoholism)* because his words were slurred.

Nurse Cathy realized that Elsa was dependent on Mark and in a vulnerable situation and that Mark, who also had risk factors, was also in a vulnerable situation. She sensed that providing Elsa with home care and postrehabilitation services may not be enough and that additional services such as counseling were needed to prevent the situation from escalating into actual abuse. Nurse Cathy requested that Bonnie, a BRIA social worker, become involved.

SOCIAL WORKER BONNIE: ASSESSING THE OVERALL SITUATION AND USING THE RISK OF ABUSE TOOL WITH NURSE CATHY

Social Worker Bonnie arranged her initial visit at a time when she could talk privately to Elsa. During this home visit, Elsa broke down and confided in Bonnie. Bonnie learned the details of Elsa's life and realized that she held strong and traditional values, was proud of her role as a mother, and loved her son dearly. Elsa wept as she told Bonnie that she felt she had failed her husband, Joseph, after his death because she could not raise an ideal son. She recounted Mark's history of work-related problems and his issues with alcoholism. She could not understand why Mark spent days in his room, appeared so downhearted, and sometimes got angry about small things. To determine the risk of abuse occurring in the future, Bonnie and Nurse Cathy reviewed the situation and checked off risk factors pertaining to Elsa and Mark from the Risk of Abuse Tool, as illustrated in Figure 10.1.

CARE PLAN DEVELOPED FOR ELSA AND MARK: DESCRIBING THE TEAM APPROACH TO PREVENTING ABUSE

Nurse Cathy, Social Worker Bonnie, and one of the BRIA mental health case managers developed a comprehensive plan of care to address both the physical and psychosocial needs of Elsa and Mark. Nurse Cathy and Social Worker Bonnie visited to discuss the components of the plan and gain Elsa's and Mark's consent. Initially, Elsa was overwhelmed by the plan of care, but she eventually began to trust the BRIA team and accepted the plan as it evolved. The plan gradually moved from home health services, nursing, and physical therapy to include counseling, mental health services for her hoarding behavior, home-delivered meals to help her get nutritious meals, and attending an adult day-care program to meet her socialization needs. At every step, Elsa provided input about her personal preferences with regard to when and how much help she wanted. Elsa gradually convinced Mark to discuss his situation with the team so he could become independent and provide for himself. Table 14.1 delineates the issues, interventions, and outcomes of the plan implemented by the team.

SUMMARY

The case presented in this chapter demonstrates how a community-based agency, particularly its home health care department, supported and expanded the role of the nurse to address not only the medical issues, but also the vulnerabilities that made the older adult susceptible to abuse. The nurse involved in the case was able to involve a multidisciplinary team to formulate a comprehensive plan of care that addressed risks in both the older adult and the caregiver. The nurse

TABLE 14.1 Benjamin Rose Institute on Aging Plan of Care for Client and Caregiver

KEY ISSUES FOR ELSA AND MARK	RECOMMENDED INTERVENTIONS	OUTCOMES
Home environment needs modifications.	The nurse recommends adding outside railings, grab bars, shower chair, and a raised toilet seat.	All modifications are done.
Elsa needs assistance with activities of daily living.	A home health aide will help with bathing, dressing, and grooming three times weekly for 6 weeks.	Elsa receives needed care when home health aide is there.
Elsa's mobility is limited and unsafe.	Physical therapy visits will occur twice weekly for 6 weeks.	Elsa progresses to safe ambulation with walker.
Neither Elsa nor Mark are knowledgeable about wound care.	Skilled nursing is provided for assessment, treatment, and education about wound care.	Incision heals without complications.
Lack of understanding about diabetes management.	Skilled nursing is provided for teaching about diabetes self-management.	Elsa achieves better management of diabetes.
Both Elsa and Mark have mental health needs.	The nurse obtains the physician's order for skilled social worker care.	Social worker becomes involved.
Elsa expresses significant anxiety related to her perceived failure as a mother and strong beliefs in strict gender roles.	The social worker provides skilled counseling, once or twice weekly, for 6 weeks; he or she also identifies and addresses the sources of Elsa's anxiety.	Elsa becomes less anxious and improves in self-esteem.
Elsa is dependent on Mark for meal preparation; Mark is reluctant to help.	Home-delivered meals are provided for Elsa.	Elsa's diabetes is managed and nutritional needs are met; Mark is less anxious.

(continued)

TABLE 14.1 Benjamin Rose Institute on Aging Plan of Care for Client and Caregiver *(continued)*

KEY ISSUES FOR ELSA AND MARK	RECOMMENDED INTERVENTIONS	OUTCOMES
Elsa has a hoarding problem.	Mental health services address issues.	Pathways are cleared and environment is safe.
Elsa admits to social isolation.	After skilled services terminate, Elsa will attend adult day care and receive transportation services.	Elsa responds positively to social interactions; Elsa's self-esteem improves.
Mark is overwhelmed by caregiving responsibilities.	The nurse provides support and education; the social worker provides counseling and facilitates referrals.	Mark's anxiety is alleviated.
Mark uses alcohol excessively to cope with stress.	The social worker talks with Mark about Alcoholics Anonymous.	Mark agrees to attend and begins his road to recovery.
Mark is unemployed and depressed.	The social worker talks with Mark about mental health resources and facilitates a referral for county employment services.	Mark finds employment and his mental health needs are addressed.

understood that Elsa was not being abused by her son but that the situation was ripe with risk factors that could develop into an abusive situation. Thus, in addition to providing and arranging for skilled home care services, the nurse facilitated additional services and supports for Elsa, including counseling, home-delivered meals, and adult day-care services. In addition, BRIA staff supported Elsa in convincing Mark to seek help for alcoholism, depression, and unemployment. Interventions of the BRIA staff over the course of several months enabled Elsa and Mark to deal with their physical and mental health-related issues. They gained insight into their family dynamics, learned to address their issues, and eventually developed a better relationship.

KEY POINTS: WHAT NURSES NEED TO KNOW AND CAN DO

- Identify risks that increase an older adult's vulnerability to an abusive situation, such as the ones delineated in the Risk of Abuse Tool.

- Facilitate referrals for services to proactively address issues that can develop into an abusive situation.

REFERENCES

Anetzberger, G. J. (2006). *Ohio adult protective services core curriculum: Adult protective services assessment* (Unpublished report). Ohio Department of Job and Family Services, Columbus, OH.

Anetzberger, G. J., & Ejaz, F. K. (2016). *Findings from case managers participating in an online training on abuse and its reporting.* Workshop presented at the annual meeting of the American Society on Aging, Washington, DC. Retrieved from http://www.benrose.org/News/ASA-2016-Online-Training-on-Abuse.pdf

Bass, D. M., Anetzberger, G. J., Ejaz, F. K., & Nagpaul, K. (2001). Screening tools and referral protocol for stopping abuse against older Ohioans: A guide for service providers. *Journal of Elder Abuse & Neglect, 13*(2), 23–38.

Benjamin Rose Institute on Aging (BRIA). (n.d.). *Services of the Benjamin Rose Institute on Aging.* Retrieved from http://www.benrose.org

Ejaz, F. K., Bass, D. M., Anetzberger, G. J., & Nagpaul, K. (2001). Evaluating the Ohio elder abuse and domestic violence in late life screening tools and referral protocol. *Journal of Elder Abuse & Neglect, 13*, 39–57.

Ejaz, F. K., Bukach, A., Conway, A., & Anetzberger, G. J. (2014, October). *Development of online training modules on abuse, neglect, and exploitation for care managers in MyCare Ohio.* (Unpublished report to Ohio Department of Aging and the Administration for Community Living). Benjamin Rose Institute on Aging, Cleveland, OH. Retrieved from http://www.benrose.org/education/odadevelopment.pdf

BENJAMIN ROSE INSTITUTE ON AGING (BRIA)

Acknowledgments. The authors would like to thank the Ohio Department of Aging (ODA) for funding the development, testing, and implementation of an online training program on abuse, neglect, and exploitation from a larger initiative supported by the U.S. Administration for Community Living; Karla Warren, Program Officer at ODA; Dr. Georgia Anetzberger, project consultant; other team members at

BRIA who were involved in the development, testing, and/or implementation of the training: Ashley Bukach, Alycia Conway, Mahum Abbas, and Zishan Arooj; and Advisory Council members and other professionals who helped test the training and its products. We would also like to thank Miriam Rose, Senior Research Analyst, for editorial assistance.

For more information, please contact the primary author, Dr. Farida K. Ejaz, at: fejaz@benrose.org or 216-373-1660. The Risk of Abuse Tool is copyrighted by the Benjamin Rose Institute on Aging. For use of the tool for noncommercial purposes, please refer to Ejaz et al. (2014; available at www.benrose.org). *Development of Online Training Modules on Abuse, Neglect, and Exploitation for Care Managers in MyCare Ohio.* (Unpublished report to Ohio Department of Aging and the Administration for Community Living.) Benjamin Rose Institute on Aging, Cleveland, Ohio (will be available at www.benrose.org).

THE NURSE'S GUIDE TO FINANCIAL ABUSE AND SEXUAL ABUSE OF OLDER ADULTS

FINANCIAL ABUSE OF OLDER ADULTS IN ITS MANY FORMS AND GUISES

Financial abuse (also called exploitation) is the illegal or improper use of an elder's funds, property, or assets. Examples range from seemingly harmless and minor incidents to outright criminal acquisition of significant assets or property of an older adult, as described in the next section. Several studies cite financial abuse as the type of elder abuse that occurs most commonly, accounting for 30% to 50% of cases in domestic settings (Metlife Mature Market Institute, 2009; National Center on Elder Abuse, 1998). Prevalence studies indicate that between 3.5% and 5% of community-dwelling older adults—presumably with relatively high levels of functioning—told interviewers that they had experienced at least one episode of financial abuse during the previous year (Acierno, Hernandez-Tejada, Muzzy, & Steve, 2009; Lauman, Leitsch, & Waite, 2008; Lifespan of Greater Rochester, Weill Cornell Medical Center, & the State of New York Department of Aging, 2011). These statistics do not include unreported cases or financial abuse of older adults who reside in long-term care facilities.

Recently, financial abuse has been gaining public attention as an issue that needs to be addressed at many levels, including by health care professionals. An analysis of data from one of the largest and most methodologically rigorous studies of elder abuse concluded that financial abuse of older adults is a public health crisis that merits the attention of clinicians, policy makers, researchers, and any citizen who cares about the dignity and well-being of older Americans (Peterson et al., 2014.)

WHAT WE KNOW ABOUT FINANCIAL ABUSE

Financial abuse of older adults is a complex phenomenon that occurs as a single type of abuse or in combination with other types, such as physical or psychological abuse. Similarly, older adults may be victims of financial abuse only once or twice or they may experience it intermittently or over the long term. Examples of some of the many ways in which older adults experience financial abuse are as follows:

- Paid caregivers "stealing time" by engaging in personal activities while being paid to provide care and ignoring the needs of the person who pays them

- Trusted others who control assets of older adults and use them for their own benefit and without consent (e.g., using undue influence to transfer deeds to property or titles to vehicles)

- Trusted others or strangers who use the older adult's credit card without authorization or permission

- Trusted others who acquire assets by enticing an older adult to sign deeds, retirement accounts, or other legal documents without the capacity to understand the action

- Trusted others or strangers who forge an older person's signature for financial gain

- Improper use of conservatorship, guardianship, or power of attorney

- Family members with addictions who take money or property to support their habits

- Predatory lenders who pressure older homeowners to take out home equity loans at exorbitant rates or with unfair terms

- Scammers—or even well-intentioned people—who charm or romance an older adult with the intent of using the person's assets and then abandon him or her after the assets are acquired and care is needed

- Unscrupulous home repair people who do not provide the services they are paid to do

- Scammers who solicit money under false pretenses and take advantage of older adults who are lonely, vulnerable, gullible, or cognitively impaired

- Identity theft by paid caregivers and nursing home employees

As illustrated in these examples, perpetrators include trusted professionals, adult children, family, friends, neighbors, strangers, and even criminals. Perpetrators' motives vary widely and include greed, desperation, retribution, and expectations. Not all perpetrators understand that their actions are illegal and immoral, for example, when a family member manages an older adult's finances and does not understand that money should be spent only for the older person. In some situations, cultural norms or unclear agreements about compensation for caregiving can make it difficult to define financial abuse.

Conditions most consistently cited as risks for financial abuse are female sex, dependency, and increased age (i.e., between 70 and 89 years). A recent study of 4,156 community-living adults age 60 or older concluded that risk for financial abuse is associated with "a distinct and all too familiar profile of social and economic vulnerability in the United States." Included in this description are older adults who (a) are African Americans, (b) have incomes that are below the poverty line, (c) are dependent on others for care, and (d) reside in households with nonspousal members (Peterson et al., 2014, p. 1621). Similarly, a study by Beach and colleagues (2010) found that the 6-month prevalence of financial exploitation was nearly six times greater for African Americans compared with non-African Americans.

The most obvious consequence of financial abuse is loss of money, which can be significant. Interviews with 71 adult protective service workers and their clients in Virginia found that 88.7% of the clients experienced adverse financial consequences with an average loss of $87,967 and only 16% receiving any restitution (Jackson & Hafemeister, 2010). Among the psychosocial consequences are negative effects on personal relationships, conflicts among family members, and feelings such as anger, shame, self-blame, and resentment.

Although financial abuse is typically associated with legal or criminal matters, it is less obviously—but just as importantly—related to the health of older adults in the following ways:

- Health conditions, such as impaired cognition, physical disability, or mental health issues, can increase the risk for financial abuse.

- Financial abuse depletes the older adult's income and assets and diminishes their ability to pay for medications, medical supplies, health care, and other health-related needs.

- The ability to manage—and protect—one's money and assets is an instrumental activity of daily living (IADL) that needs to be assessed within the context of safe and independent functioning.

Professional publications discuss the essential roles of primary care practitioners and other health care clinicians in recognizing and addressing financial abuse of older adults in clinical settings (e.g., Factora, 2014; Fitzwater & Puchta, 2010). The following sections of this chapter describe ways in which nurses can identify and address financial abuse when they care for older adults. Case examples illustrate application of this information to clinical settings. The testimony of Mickey Rooney for the Senate Special Committee on Aging (Case 15.1) illustrates many of the points discussed in this chapter.

CASE 15.1 Testimony of Mickey Rooney for the Senate Special Committee on Aging, March 2, 2011

Throughout my life, I have been blessed with the love and support of family, friends, and fans. I have worked almost my entire lifetime of 90 years to entertain and please other people. I've worked hard and diligently. But even with this success, my money was stolen from me, by someone close. I was unable to avoid becoming a victim of elder abuse.

Elder abuse comes in many different forms—physical abuse, emotional abuse, or financial abuse. Each one is devastating in its own right. Many times, sadly, as with my situation, the elder abuse involves a family member. When that happens, you feel scared, disappointed, angry, and you can't believe this is happening to you. You feel overwhelmed. The strength you need to fight it is complicated. You're afraid, but you're also thinking about your other family members. You're thinking about the potential criticism of your family and friends. They may not want to accept the dysfunction that you need to share. Because you love your family and for other reasons, you might feel hesitant to come forward. You might not be able to make rational decisions. What other people see as generosity may, in reality, be the exploitation, manipulation, and sadly, emotional blackmail of older, more vulnerable members of the American public.

I know because it happened to me. My money was taken and misused. When I asked for information, I was told that I couldn't have any of my own information. I was told it was "for my own good" and that "it was none of my business." I was literally left powerless.

(continued)

CASE 15.1 Testimony of Mickey Rooney for the Senate Special Committee on Aging, March 2, 2011 *(continued)*

You can be in control of your life one minute and in the next minute, you have absolutely no control. Sometimes this happens quickly, but other times it is very gradual. You wonder when it truly began. In my case, I was eventually and completely stripped of the ability to make even the most basic decisions in my own life.

Over the course of time, my daily life became unbearable. Worse, it seemed to happen out of nowhere. At first, it was something small, something I could control. But then it became something sinister that was completely out of control. I felt trapped, scared, used, and frustrated. But above all, I felt helpless. For years I suffered silently. I couldn't muster the courage to seek the help I knew I needed. Even when I tried to speak up, I was told to be quiet. It seemed like no one believed me. But I never gave up. I continued to share my story with others. . . . If elder abuse happened to me, Mickey Rooney, it can happen to anyone. Myself, who I am, what I hope to be, and what I was, was taken from me.

Nursing Reflections on Mickey Rooney's Situation

Mickey Rooney's situation is very real and sad and contains lessons for nurses. He depended on his grandson for care and he was abused psychologically and financially—perhaps even in other ways. In addition to the significant loss of assets, he experienced serious emotional consequences. Despite Mickey Rooney's fears, distress, and feelings of helplessness, he eventually sought resolution of his abusive situation. He testified that he suffered silently for years before he found the courage to come forward and seek help.

As a nurse, I wonder how many encounters Mickey Rooney had with health care professionals while he was being abused. I wonder if his grandson accompanied him to health care appointments. I wonder if any health care professionals made efforts to ask him in private about any concerns he might have had. I wonder if he sought opportunities to confide in health care professionals but was ignored. I wonder if I would have been able to help Mickey Rooney if I provided care for him when he was being abused. I hope I learn from his story and recognize the indicators when I care for older adults who may be in abusive situations.

RESPONSIBILITIES OF NURSES RELATED TO IDENTIFYING AND REPORTING FINANCIAL ABUSE

As with other aspects of elder abuse, nurses are responsible for identifying indicators, assessing the overall situation, and reporting suspected cases of financial abuse. Identification of financial abuse is hampered by barriers that are similar to those inherent in other elder abuse situations, such as the victim's feelings of shame or helplessness, or the person's dependency on or fear of the perpetrator. Barriers that are more specific to financial abuse include the following:

- Lack of access to information that provides evidence of or clues to financial abuse
- Perception that it is too late to do anything about it
- Fear that exposure of exploitation will lead to appointment of a guardian or conservator
- Desire to protect a trusted other from legal or criminal actions

An older adult can experience financial abuse once, occasionally, or frequently over months or years. Many times, it is well hidden and discovered only afterward, especially when it is not ongoing or when the perpetrator is highly motivated to hide any evidence. In some situations, especially when the perpetrator is a trusted other, financial abuse may be part of a larger pattern of abuse that includes other types. Thus, nurses need to identify risks for and indicators of financial abuse and consider the clues in the context of the overall situation. Box 15.1 delineates indicators that should raise the suspicion of financial abuse.

As with all situations of suspected abuse, nurses need to build a trusting relationship and seek additional information so they can assess the broader situation. Additional clues are sometimes found in the context of the older adult's health-related needs. For example, when financial abuse is ongoing or when the older adult's assets have been depleted, the nurse may observe indicators such as any of the following: nonadherence to medications, worsening medical conditions, missed appointments, anxiety, depression, decline in functioning, or a change in behavior. As with other types of elder abuse, when nurses suspect that financial abuse is occurring or has occurred, they need to report to appropriate agencies, such as adult protective services, as illustrated in Case 15.2.

BOX 15.1 Guide to Identifying Indicators of Financial Abuse

Red flags indicative of financial abuse

- Sudden changes in bank account or banking practice
- An unexplained withdrawal of large sums of money, particularly if an older adult is accompanied during financial transactions by someone else
- Unexplained inclusion of additional names on an elder's bank account
- Unauthorized withdrawal of the elder's funds using the elder's ATM card
- Abrupt changes in a will or other financial documents
- Unexplained disappearance of funds or valuable possessions
- Substandard care being provided or bills unpaid despite the availability of adequate financial resources
- Discovery of an elder's signature being forged for financial transactions or for the titles of his or her possessions
- Sudden appearance of previously uninvolved relatives claiming their rights to an elder's affairs and possessions
- Unexplained sudden transfer of assets to a family member or someone outside the family
- The provision of services that are not necessary
- The older adult's report of financial exploitation or questionable transactions

CASE 15.2 Visiting Nurse Identifies and Reports Financial Abuse

Gertrude still lives in the home in which she was born 86 years ago, in a rural county in the Midwest. Gertrude has been hospitalized several times during the last year for unstable heart failure and she now receives skilled nursing care. During Nurse Samantha's first visit, Gertrude said she was ashamed of the run-down condition of her house, stating she had been in and out of the hospital so much she could never follow through with plans for repairs. Nurse Samantha noted that buckets were placed in several rooms to catch the water from leaks in the ceilings. Windows were old and did not close tightly and the water was turned off to the tub.

(continued)

CASE 15.2 Visiting Nurse Identifies and Reports Financial Abuse
(continued)

Gertrude told Nurse Samantha that "a nice young man—I think his name was Bill—stopped by a couple months ago and said he was certified by the county office on aging to do home repair work. He told me he was a good friend of Susan, the person who delivers my meals on wheels. He even told me about a special fund that the office on aging has to pay for home repairs for senior citizens who have lived in their homes for at least 25 years. I gave him a check for $5,000 so he could buy new windows and the materials for the roof and he said he'd help me get reimbursed from the special fund. Well, I gave him a check and then ended up in the hospital and he hasn't come around again. He didn't leave a phone number, but he told me I could get in touch with him through Susan, so I'll ask her about him the next time I see her."

During each of the next four visits, Nurse Samantha asked Gertrude about any success with getting contact information for Bill. Each time Gertrude said she kept forgetting to ask Susan, but she was confident that Bill would be bringing the windows as soon as the weather got warmer. During Nurse Samantha's fifth visit, Susan was delivering Gertrude's meal and Nurse Samantha reminded Gertrude to ask about Bill. Susan declared, "Oh no, I never heard of Bill until a couple of the people on my delivery route asked me if I knew him. When I asked Paul, our center director, about this he told me that a man named Bill used to work in the maintenance department but was fired about 8 months ago. I guess Bill got to know the names of all of us who work out of the center. You could call Paul to find out what he knows about Bill."

After calling Paul from Gertrude's house, Nurse Samantha finds out that several older adults in the county have asked about Bill but none of the others has given him any money. Nurse Samantha calls the county adult protective services agency from Gertrude's house and is told that this is not an isolated episode and they will visit Gertrude so they can begin an investigation.

RESPONSIBILITIES OF NURSES RELATED TO ASSESSMENT OF FINANCIAL CAPACITY

The concept of financial capacity is integral to the topic of financial abuse, particularly in relation to responsibilities of health care professionals. Financial capacity is defined as the ability to independently manage one's financial affairs in a manner that is consistent with one's values and self-interest (Marson, 2013). An individual's financial capacity affects numerous daily and intermittent activities, ranging from small transactions such as shopping and bill paying to major transactions that have long-term and often irreversible consequences (e.g., selling or purchasing property, signing legal documents). Assessment of financial capacity is pertinent to elder abuse in the following ways:

- Financial capacity is an essential skill for safe and independent functioning.

- Diminished financial capacity increases the risk for elder abuse, scams, and financial exploitation.

- Diminished financial capacity is one of the earliest clinical signs of an emerging dementia.

- Loss of financial capacity can be psychologically distressing.

- Assessment of financial capacity is associated with legal and ethical implications with regard to respecting autonomy versus appointing someone to manage the person's finances.

- When issues related to diminished financial capacity are not addressed, older adults are at risk for significant financial losses.

- Inability to manage finances is strongly associated with increased burden and time demands for family caregivers.

- When diminished financial capacity increases the older adult's risk for exploitation and abuse, clinicians may be morally and legally responsible for reporting. (Marson, 2013; Razani et al., 2007; Widera, Steenpass, Marson, & Sudore, 2011).

Recent articles in professional journals discuss the assessment of financial capacity as a professional responsibility of all health care providers who are required to report elder abuse (e.g., Caboral-Stevens & Medetsky, 2014; Flint, Sudore, & Widera, 2012).

Health care professionals consider financial capacity in the context of assessing IADL along with other complex activities such as meal preparation, grocery shopping, use of telephone, and medication management. In the context of elder abuse, nurses assess IADL so interventions can be initiated to improve safety and functioning, as discussed in Chapters 9 and 10. For example, nurses routinely assess IADL related to the ability of older adults to meet their nutritional needs or adhere to medication routines. This same approach applies to assessing an older adult's ability to protect his or her assets, and, in fact, is necessary for identifying interventions that may be effective in preventing financial abuse.

Nurses are not responsible for assessing an older adult's financial capacity, but they are responsible for identifying the need for such an assessment and facilitating referrals when the need is identified. It is important to note that some of the evidence is based on identifying behaviors that reflect a decline in the older adult's baseline level of financial functioning. Additional evidence is gathered through direct clinical assessments and through discussion with older adults and their families and caregivers, but with precautions such as the following:

- Older adults may not have insight into or be aware of their cognitive deficits.
- Older adults may try to cover up their cognitive deficits.
- Families or caregivers may purposefully provide inaccurate information so they can gain control over the older adult's assets.

Nurses can use Box 15.2 to identify indicators of the need for assessment of financial capacity.

Facilitating Referrals for Assessment of Financial Capacity

Assessment of financial capacity (sometimes called financial decision-making capacity) is evolving as an area of specialization within the domain of geriatrics, with formal assessment tools currently being evaluated. A comprehensive assessment of financial capacity considers the following components: contextual factors, usual cognitive functioning, and consistency of current behaviors with the person's values, as illustrated in Figure 15.1. Although specialized resources for assessment of financial capacity are limited, nurses can suggest or initiate a referral to a comprehensive geriatric assessment program (as described in Chapter 11). Case 15.3 describes a situation in which a nurse practitioner addresses the need for a financial capacity assessment.

NURSING INTERVENTIONS FOR PREVENTING FINANCIAL ABUSE

Nurses have important roles in teaching older adults and family members about interventions to protect the older adult's assets and prevent financial abuse. Adult children are likely to overestimate their parents' ability to manage their finances, avoid using formal mechanisms (e.g., power of attorney documents), and "tend to think of their parents'

BOX 15.2 Guide to Identifying the Need for Assessment of Financial Capacity

Behaviors that reflect a decline in the person's baseline level of financial functioning
- Increasing memory lapses that affect one's ability to fulfill financial obligations (e.g., not paying bills, forgetting how to write a check)
- Increasing disorganization of financial or legal documents (e.g., misplacing important documents, failing to perform mandatory withdrawals from retirement accounts)
- Decline in ability to manage checking account (e.g., failing to enter information in check register)
- Decline in mathematical skills (e.g., new problems with written or oral arithmetic)
- Loss of general knowledge about basic financial terms, such as mortgage, legal documents, or investments
- Diminished judgment about investments or money management
- New and abiding interest in get-rich-quick schemes
- Unfounded anxiety about the nature and extent of one's personal wealth

Evidence from clinical assessments
- Diagnosis of medical condition that may affect cognition or functional ability (i.e., mild cognitive impairment, dementia, stroke)
- Impairments identified in basic cognitive tests
- Noticeable changes in hygiene, behavior, or appearance
- Loss of partner or other person who had been managing finances
- Unfamiliar family members or caregivers accompanying patient to clinic visit

Evidence based on reports of patients, families, or caregivers
- Recent onset of difficulty paying for medications or basic necessities
- Notices about disconnection of utilities or eviction from apartment
- Confusion about assets or bank accounts (e.g., thinking that funds are missing)
- Erratic, unusual, or uncharacteristic purchases, withdrawals, or gifts
- Accusations that others are stealing or mismanaging one's funds
- Disclosure of new and dubious relationships

Adapted from Widera et al. (2011).

FIGURE 15.1 Components of the financial decisional abilities model.

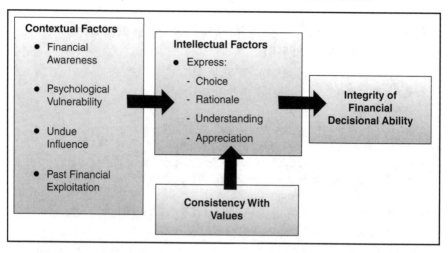

Source: Lichtenberg, Stoltman, Ficker, Iris, and Mast (2015). Adapted with permission of Haworth Press, Inc. via Copyright Clearance Center. (Taylor & Francis Ltd, http://www.tandfonline.com).

CASE 15.3 Nurse Practitioner Refers a Patient for Financial Capacity Assessment

Jacqueline, who is 75 years old, lives alone and views herself as healthy. She volunteers at the library and enjoys attending the local senior center for social activities. Jacqueline sees her nurse practitioner every 2 months for management of chronic conditions, including arthritis, type 2 diabetes, and coronary artery disease. Usually, Jacqueline is very punctual and she calls in a timely manner when she needs to change an appointment, but 2 weeks ago, Jacqueline missed her regular appointment and today she was an hour late. Nurse Practitioner Cecelia asks Jacqueline if she is having any difficulty with any of her usual activities, like managing her medications or paying bills. Jacqueline admits that she missed payments on a few bills and was surprised when she recently received a shut-off notice for her electricity. Nurse Practitioner Cecelia tells Jacqueline she is concerned about these changes and wants to make sure that she remains as independent as possible. She refers Jacqueline to the comprehensive geriatric assessment program and emphasizes that the staff can identify underlying causes. They will also help Jacqueline find reliable resources for managing medications, bill paying, and other important activities while supporting Jacqueline's desire to be independent.

assets as 'almost theirs'" (Mukherjee, 2013, p. 425). When deficits in financial capacity are identified, interventions are directed toward protecting assets while at the same time respecting the person's autonomy. Even when older adults have full financial capacity, preventive measures are usually appropriate. For example, a legal document appointing a trustworthy person as an attorney-in-fact (also called durable power of attorney) for financial affairs can help protect one's assets from financial abuse. This document takes effect only after the person has been deemed to lack capacity, and it can grant global financial authority or restrict authority to certain transactions.

Simple measures such as automatic deposits, bill paying, overdraft protection, notifying a third party if bills are not paid, and joint bank accounts with a trustworthy person are useful in many situations. Nurses have opportunities to teach older adults and their families about these preventive measures, as illustrated in Case 15.4. When

---

CASE 15.4 Nurse in Acute Care Setting Teaches Older Adult About Measures for Protecting Financial Assets

Nurse Liam is preparing Anthony, who is 73 years old, for discharge to his home following a hospitalization for pneumonia. Anthony has macular degeneration, but otherwise is healthy; the only medication he took before being hospitalized is Ocuvite. He uses low-vision aids at home and participates in social activities at the local senior center. Nurse Liam asks Anthony what kind of assistance he receives at home, and is told that a neighbor, Brenda, has been visiting two times a week to prepare meals, provide transportation, and assist with laundry and housekeeping. Anthony says that Brenda will be coming more often after he gets home because he will need additional help, especially with managing his new medications. Anthony also says that Brenda has offered to come more often so she can assist with his banking and bill paying because his eyesight seems to be worsening.

Anthony's daughter, Angela, is present for the discharge discussion and she expresses surprise and concern about Brenda's offer. She tells Nurse Liam that she had accompanied her father to an eye doctor appointment 2 weeks ago and the examination did not show any progression. Angela lives 250 miles away, but she visits at least monthly, even though Anthony reports that he gets along fine with Brenda's help. Angela

(continued)

CASE 15.4 Nurse in Acute Care Setting Teaches Older Adult About Measures for Protecting Financial Assets *(continued)*

states that she worries that Brenda will take advantage of her father's loneliness, as well as his significant financial assets. Anthony says that having Brenda write checks would be convenient but he, too, has questions about her trustworthiness. He trusts Angela totally but he does not want to bother her with bill paying when she visits.

Nurse Liam suggests that Anthony and Angela work together to implement the following measures to avoid the need for Brenda to become involved and to protect Anthony's assets from potential exploitation: (a) Establish a new joint checking account with online bill paying, which would be done by Angela; (b) maintain enough balance in the checking account to cover monthly expenses but keep large amounts of money in other accounts; (c) keep all financial documents; (d) meet with Anthony's usual financial planner to establish measures.

discussing these measures with older adults, it is imperative to address their wishes for privacy and independence, while at the same time providing an appropriate level of support and protection. It is also important to recognize that these issues need to be addressed periodically based on the changing needs and health status of the older adult.

RESOURCES FOR ADDRESSING FINANCIAL ABUSE

Increasing attention to financial abuse has led to the development of coalitions involving groups from many sectors, such as consumer organizations, nonprofit agencies, and all levels of government. For example, many states have established financial abuse programs under their Attorney General's offices. In addition, agencies that historically have addressed elder abuse (e.g., adult protective services and Long-Term Care Ombudsman) are developing specialized services focusing on financial abuse, such as financial abuse specialist teams (FAST). Box 15.3 identifies some of the resources for professional and consumer information about financial abuse that were available in 2016. Nurses can find up-to-date information about additional resources by contacting state agencies listed in the appendices of this book.

BOX 15.3 Financial Abuse Prevention Programs

Consumer Financial Protection Bureau, www.consumerfinance.gov
- *Money Smart for Older Adults,* consumer education course about prevention of financial abuse, avoidance of scams, and protection of one's assets

Elder Investment Fraud and Financial Exploitation (EIFFE) Prevention Program, www.nasaa.org/1733/eiffe/
- Major collaborative effort to educate medical professionals who care for older adults about how to refer at-risk older adults to the appropriate authorities
- Online printable resources for professionals and consumers (e.g., *Clinician's Pocket Guide, Senior Patient Education Brochure*)

National Center on Elder Abuse, www.ncea.aoa.gov
- Information for professionals and educational brochures for older adults

National Committee for Prevention of Elder Abuse, www.preventeldera buse.org
- Information for professionals

Examples of state coalitions to address financial abuse
- California: Elder Financial Protection Network, www.elderfinancial protection.org
- Florida: Protect Yourself From Financial Exploitation, http://edleraffairs .state.fl.us/does/abuse_prevention.php
- New York: New York State Coalition on Elder Abuse, Resources on Financial Abuse, http://nyelderabuse.org

KEY POINTS: WHAT NURSES NEED TO KNOW AND CAN DO

- Much research indicates that financial abuse is the type of abuse that occurs most commonly but is the least reported.
- Although any older adult can become a victim of financial abuse, conditions that are associated with being at risk include female sex, dependency, increased age, and African American race.
- Nurses are responsible for identifying risks (Box 15.1) and reporting suspected cases.

- Health care practitioners, including nurses, have important roles in identifying the need for assessment of financial capacity (Box 15.2) and facilitating referrals when the need is identified (Case 15.3).

- Nurses can teach older adults and their families about interventions to prevent financial abuse (Box 15.3).

REFERENCES

Acierno, R., Hernandez-Tejada, M., Muzzy, W., & Steve, K. (2009). *National Elder Mistreatment Study*. Report to the National Institute of Justice (Project #2007-WG-BX-0009). Rockville, MD: National Institute of Justice.

Beach, S. R., Schulz, R., Castle, N. G., & Rosen, J. (2010). Financial exploitation and psychological mistreatment among older adults: Differences between African Americans and non-African Americans in a population-based survey. *Gerontologist, 50*, 744–757.

Caboral-Stevens, M., & Medetsky, M. (2014). The construct of financial capacity in older adults. *Journal of Gerontological Nursing, 40*(8), 30–37.

Factora, R. M. (Ed). (2014). *Aging and money: Reducing risk of financial exploitation and protecting financial resources*. New York, NY: Humana Press.

Fitzwater, E., & Puchta, C. (2010). Elder abuse and financial exploitation: Unlawful and just plain awful! *Journal of Gerontological Nursing, 16*(12), 3–5.

Flint, L. A., Sudore, R. L., & Widera, E. (2012). Assessing financial capacity impairment in older adults. *Generations, 36*, 59–65.

Jackson, S. L., & Hafemeister, T. L. (2010). *Financial abuse of elderly people vs other forms of elder abuse: Assessing their dynamics, risk factors, and society's response: Final report to the National Institute of Justice*. Washington, DC: National Institute of Justice, U.S. Department of Justice.

Lauman, E. O., Leitsch, S., & Waite, L. (2008). Elder mistreatment in the United States. *Journal of Gerontology: Psychological and Social Sciences, 63*, S248–S254.

Lichtenberg, P. A., Stoltman, J., Ficker, L. J., Iris, M., & Mast, B. (2015). A person-centered approach to financial capacity assessment: Preliminary development of a new rating scale. *Clinical Gerontologist, 38*, 49–67.

Lifespan of Greater Rochester, Weill Cornell Medical Center, & the State of New York Department of Aging. (2011). *Under the radar: New York State Elder Abuse Prevalence Study*. Retrieved at www.lifespan-roch.org

Marson, D. C. (2013). Clinical and ethical aspects of financial capacity in dementia. *American Journal of Geriatric Psychiatry, 21*(4), 382–390.

Metlife Mature Market Institute. (2009). *Broken trust: Elders, family, and finances*. Westport, CT: Author.

Mukherjee, D. (2013). Financial exploitation of older adults in rural settings: A family perspective. *Journal of Elder Abuse & Neglect, 25*, 425–437.

National Center on Elder Abuse. (1998). *National Elder Abuse Incidence Study: Final report.* Washington, DC: National Center on Elder Abuse at the American Public Welfare Association.

Peterson, J. C., Burnes, D., Caccamise, P., Mason, A., Henderson, C., Wells, M. T., . . . Lachs, M. S. (2014). Financial exploitation of older adults: A population-based prevalence study. *Journal of General Internal Medicine, 29,* 1615–1623.

Razani, J., Kakos, B., Orieta-Barbalace, C., Wong, J. T., Casas, R., Lu, P. . . . Josephson, K. (2007). Predicting caregiver burden from daily functional abilities of patients with mild dementia. *Journal of the American Geriatrics Society, 55,* 1415–1420.

Rooney, M. (2011). *Testimony of Mickey Rooney, Senate Special Committee on Aging, March 2, 2011.* Washington, DC: U.S. Senate Special Committee on Aging.

Widera, E., Steenpass, V., Marson, D., & Sudore, R. (2011). Finances in the older patient with cognitive impairment: He didn't want me to take over. *Journal of the American Geriatrics Society, 305,* 698–706.

SEXUAL ABUSE OF OLDER ADULTS IN ITS MANY FORMS AND GUISES

Sexual abuse of older adults encompasses a wide array of actions, ranging from the unwanted exposure to sexually oriented jokes—perhaps viewed as seemingly harmless—to rape and other forms of serious sexual assault. Of all types of elder abuse, sexual abuse is the most difficult to discuss, but in many ways it is also the most important type because of its invisibility as well as its serious and sometimes fatal consequences. Nurses and other health care professionals are often unaware of situations of sexual abuse, particularly in older adults. If physical sexual abuse situations are discovered, they may be addressed by forensic specialists or—as is more likely—not addressed at all. Situations of sexual abuse that do not involve assault are even more likely to be overlooked or not even recognized. With the exception of nurses who specialize in trauma care or sexual abuse, nurses in clinical settings may think they do not encounter situations of sexual abuse in older adults. In reality, however, nurses caring for older adults in any setting are likely to provide care—at least occasionally—for older adults who are victims of some type of sexual abuse.

Despite the temptation to ignore sexual abuse in a book for nurses, this chapter is included because nurses are in key positions to become confidantes for older adults who are in need of help in dealing with their situations of sexual abuse. However, before they can become confidantes, nurses need to have a base of knowledge about sexual abuse of older adults. Moreover, when indicators of sexual abuse are identified, nurses need to take action to address the situation. Of all aspects of elder abuse, nurses and other health care professionals are least prepared to recognize and address sexual abuse.

The chapter presents an overview of sexual abuse of older adults, based on current, although scant, research on the topic. It also provides evidence-based information to challenge some of the misconceptions associated with the sexual abuse of older adults. Unique aspects of nursing assessment of sexual abuse are discussed, including a guide to determining whether older adults who are cognitively impaired have the ability to consent, because this is questioned in some situations. Nursing responsibilities, which are discussed in relation to actual cases, focus on making appropriate reports and initiating referrals to appropriate resources.

OVERVIEW

The National Center on Elder Abuse (2007) defines *sexual abuse* as "non-consenting sexual contact of any kind." This definition includes a wide range of behaviors, as delineated in Box 16.1. Although the topic of sexual abuse of older adults was recognized as an aspect of domestic violence in the 1970s, until recently this subject has not had much attention in research, practice, and policy making. Between 1991 and 2008, studies revealed that some older adults are victims of sexual abuse in domestic and long-term care settings and that acts are committed by family members, paid caregivers, and other residents in facilities. Since 2010, governmental and nonprofit agencies have focused on elder sexual abuse, as discussed in Resources for Addressing Sexual Abuse of Older Adults section. Box 16.1 presents information about what is currently known about the sexual abuse of older adults.

MISCONCEPTIONS, REALITIES, AND NURSING RESPONSIBILITIES

Understanding of the sexual abuse of older adults is clouded not only by ageist biases but also by myths and misconceptions that have long been associated with sexual violence in general (e.g., that rape is a crime of passion). A nurse researcher on this topic stated this theme in

BOX 16.1 What We Know About Sexual Abuse of Older Adults

What Are the Risk Factors?

- Dependency on others combined with physical frailty and cognitive impairments (dementia in particular)
- Diminished ability to flee or resist physical attack
- Female sex, although men are also victimized
- When abused by spouse, partner, or family member, there often is a history of domestic violence or incest

Who Are the Perpetrators?

- In all settings: primarily men but woman can also be abusers
- Range in age from minors to older adults
- In community-based settings: most commonly are spouses, partners, and male relatives
- In care facilities: most commonly are other residents and facility staff
- Less likely but possible: strangers, acquaintances, visitors in facilities, online predators, and sexual predators released from prison and living in term-care facilities

What Are the Types and Examples?

Direct contact types and examples

- Fondling of breasts or genitals (e.g., while providing personal care)
- Sexualized kissing
- Harmful genital practices (e.g., invasive touching while providing peri-care to males or females)
- Actual or attempted penetration of vagina or anus (e.g., rape, attempted rape, medically unnecessary digital rectal examination)
- Oral–genital contact
- Sadistic sexual activity

(continued)

BOX 16.1   What We Know About Sexual Abuse of Older Adults (continued)

Indirect or noncontact types and examples

- Unnecessary exposure of the person's breasts or genitals (e.g., during personal care or for sexually explicit reasons)
- Provision of unwanted sexually explicit material (e.g., cartoons, cards)
- Witnessing masturbation
- Sexually explicit photography
- Forced participation in sexual discussions
- Sexual jokes or comments
- Unwanted exposure to pornography

What Are the Consequences?

- Severe psychosocial trauma, including posttraumatic stress disorder (PTSD)
- Fear, anxiety, depression, and significant changes in behavior
- Serious physical injuries, which tend to be more common and more severe in older women compared with younger women
- Increased likelihood of being admitted to a hospital
- Decline in health and functioning
- Death

a report to the U.S. Department of Justice based on data from 284 older adults who were victims of sexual abuse:

> Until relatively recently, it has been widely beyond comprehension and belief that elders could be victims of sexual assault . . . there has been a double bias in healthcare that (1) the elderly are at low risk for sexual abuse, and (2) for elders with significant cognitive disruption, it was not even possible for them to remember such an event, let alone be affected by it. (Burgess, 2006, p. 80)

Additional reasons that information about sexual abuse of older adults is limited include the following:

- It is the least researched and least reported, which may be in part because it is least common.

- Reports are often discounted or not believed.

- Evidence is frequently ignored.

- Even when it is suspected, reliable sources of evidence may be lacking.

- Even when it is reported, there may be no investigation of the perpetrator.

- Even when an investigation is initiated, the alleged perpetrator is rarely prosecuted.

Table 16.1 summarizes some of the misconceptions associated with sexual abuse of older adults, along with related accurate information found in studies and a delineation of responsibilities of nurses.

SEXUAL ABUSE OF OLDER ADULTS IN LONG-TERM CARE SETTINGS

It is not clear whether sexual abuse of older adults occurs more commonly in long-term care settings or community-based settings. However, two conclusions are clear about this topic: (a) some residents of long-term care facilities are victims of sexual abuse, and (b) nurses are the health care professionals who have direct roles in addressing sexual abuse in long-term care facilities. Sexual abuse in long-term care facilities is increasingly being addressed not only in professional literature but also by the following groups: advocacy groups, policy makers, governmental and nonprofit agencies, families of residents, and administrators and staff in long-term care facilities.

A landmark national study of characteristics of 124 residents (with mean age of 79 years) who were reported to state authorities for investigation of sexual abuse found that 48% of the alleged victims were dependent in all activities of daily living and 64% had dementia. Types of long-term care facilities in this study included nursing homes, assisted living and residential care facilities, and rehabilitation centers. The most likely perpetrator was facility staff (43%) or another resident (41%; Ramsey-Klawsnik, Teaster, Mendiondo, Marcum, & Abner, 2008). A review of literature cited in this study concluded that professional response to sexual abuse in facilities is characterized by delayed reporting, lack of thorough and timely investigations, delayed updating of registries of abusive nurse aides, inadequate involvement of law enforcement, and low rates of prosecution and conviction of offenders. Cases 16.3 and 16.4 at the end of this chapter illustrate examples of sexual

TABLE 16.1 Misconceptions, Realities, and Nursing Responsibilities Related to Sexual Abuse of Older Adults

MISUNDERSTANDINGS	REALITIES	RESPONSIBILITIES
People with dementia cannot reliably report abusive episodes.	People with dementia retain memories of emotionally based events; they can reliably report abusive episodes they have experienced or witnessed (Wiglesworth & Mosqueda, 2011).	Recognize that people with dementia may communicate through behavioral manifestations after experiencing an emotionally traumatic event
Sexual assault happens mostly to younger women.	Research has clearly revealed that sexual assault occurs at all ages and affects both men and women (Ramsey-Klawsnik, 2004; Teaster et al., 2007).	Recognize that sexual abuse has no age limits and can happen to men as well as women, particularly those who are disabled, dependent, or cognitively impaired
People with dementia experience less emotional trauma because they do not remember the event.	People with dementia who are victims of sexual abuse show the same psychosocial trauma and postabuse behavioral symptoms of distress as victims who could verbally discuss the event(s) (Burgess, Ramsey-Klawsnik, & Gregorian, 2008).	Recognize the importance of addressing consequences of sexual abuse even with older adults who cannot discuss details
Residents of care facilities are likely to have the effects of sexual assault addressed if the event is discovered.	A national study of sexual assault in care facilities found that the most commonly offered intervention among 429 victims of alleged assault was "no intervention" (Ramsey-Klawsnik, 2012).	Advocate for appropriate services for any older adult, even a person with dementia, who is a victim of sexual assault
People with dementia do not require treatment for psychological consequences after experiencing sexual abuse.	Special mental health services are needed for the sexually abused older adults, especially when there is cognitive impairment (Burgess, 2006).	Facilitate referrals for mental health services to address psychological consequences of sexual abuse

abuse in long-term care facilities along with implications for nursing interventions.

UNIQUE ASPECTS OF NURSING ASSESSMENT OF SEXUAL ABUSE

Nursing assessment of sexual abuse of older adults poses unique challenges that compound the usual difficulties associated with any elder abuse situation. Physical signs may be difficult to distinguish from age-related changes or disease-related conditions, as in the following examples: genital bruising may be attributed to rough perineal care, vaginal bleeding may be attributed to nontraumatic vaginitis, excoriated genitalia may be attributed to incontinence, or psychological manifestations may be attributed to dementia or depression. Assessment difficulties are also associated with cognitive impairment, with regard to both the collection and interpretation of information. For example, it may be difficult to determine the accuracy of the account or a report may be misinterpreted as delusional arising from dementia. These situations require astute observations of changes in behaviors, as described in Box 16.2.

It is essential to consider all indicators in the context of the broader situation and to discuss all findings with other health care providers who may have or be able to obtain additional pertinent information. An important assessment consideration for nurses in long-term care facilities is that nursing assistants and other staff or reliable observers can provide collateral information that may facilitate the identification of situations of sexual abuse.

Nursing assessment of sexual abuse is hampered by misconceptions as described in Box 16.1 and by barriers that affect the discussion and disclosure of sexual abuse such as any of the following:

- Communication limitations: impaired hearing, limited English language, neurologically based speech impairments
- Culturally based beliefs related to sexuality, roles of men and women, and marital responsibilities
- Sociocultural taboos about not discussing any issues related to sex
- Older adult's feelings of shame, embarrassment, or self-blame
- Older adult's fear of being forced to move to another setting
- Emotional, spousal, familial, or other type of personal relationship between the older adult and the perpetrator
- Older adult's dependency on the perpetrator for care or financial support

- Older adult's fear of unpleasant or harmful consequences from the perpetrator (e.g., retaliation, additional abuse)
- Older adult's lack of awareness that the conduct is sexual abuse (e.g., spousal rape)
- Actual or perceived power of the perpetrator over the older adult
- Age or gender differences between the clinician and the older adult

Although some of these barriers apply to other forms of elder abuse, these barriers add to the challenges inherent in the assessment of sexual abuse in older adults. Cultural considerations discussed in Chapter 5 and communication techniques discussed in Chapter 7 are applicable to addressing these barriers.

Nurses are not expected to investigate situations of suspected or actual sexual abuse, but they are expected to identify the need for an investigation by skilled professionals. Moreover, they are obligated to report the situation to the appropriate investigative authority, as delineated in state laws. Nurses can identify the need for an investigation by making a conscious effort to recognize direct and indirect indicators that should raise suspicion of sexual abuse. When any indicator is identified, nurses need to obtain additional information by asking questions. Box 16.2 provides a guide to nursing assessment of sexual abuse of older adults.

BOX 16.2 Guide to Nursing Assessment of Sexual Abuse

Examples of Coded Phrases That Raise Suspicion of Sexual Abuse

- "He's my boyfriend."
- "Don't let that man near me."
- "I'm his favorite girl."
- "Should I be tested for any sexual diseases?"

Physical Indicators

- Bruises to outer arms, chest, mouth, genitals, abdomen, pelvis, or inside thighs

(continued)

BOX 16.2 Guide to Nursing Assessment of Sexual Abuse *(continued)*

- Bite mark
- Torn, stained, and/or bloody bedding or clothing including underwear
- Unexplained sexually transmitted diseases or HIV

Behavioral Indicators

- Change in behavior
- Repeatedly refusing personal care
- Fear of going to sleep, nightmares
- New onset of incontinence
- Changes in appetite and eating
- Agitated or restless behavior, yelling, pacing, out-of-character disruptive behaviors
- Shock, withdrawal, staring blankly, lying in fetal position
- Depression, decreased enjoyment of social activities
- Wearing multiple layers of clothing for self-protection

Questions to Explore Sexual Abuse

- Has anyone ever touched you in your pubic area* other than when it was required for health-related reasons?
- Has anyone ever forced you to touch or look at their pubic area*?
- Has anyone touched or hugged you unnecessarily, excessively, or inappropriately while he or she is helping you with personal care or transferring?
- Has anyone ever made you undress or expose yourself when you didn't want to?
- Has anyone ever made you do anything related to your body that made you uncomfortable?
- Has anyone ever made inappropriate sexual advances and continued even when you said you did not want them?

*Use alternative terminology as appropriate (e.g. "private areas") and include breasts for women.

DIFFERENTIATING BETWEEN CONSENSUAL AND NONCONSENSUAL SEXUAL INTERACTIONS

A legal and ethical concern related to older adults who are cognitively impaired is determining whether they have the capacity to consent to sexual interactions. This issue has gained much attention from several very diverse perspectives. First, administrators and staff in long-term care facilities increasingly recognize the need to support residents' rights related to intimate and sexual relationships as a component of healthy aging and quality of life. Second, if someone who is cognitively impaired lacks the capacity to consent to sexual interactions, the behaviors may fall within the definition of sexual abuse. It is also addressed within the context of resident-to-resident abuse, which can involve one or more residents who are cognitively impaired and engage in physical sexual interactions with other residents.

Determination of capacity for consent to sexual activity may require the assessment skills of several professionals, and nurses are in key positions to identify the need for such an assessment. Nurses not only observe sexual behaviors and overall functioning of residents, but they also hear questions from staff, other residents, families, and guardians about the appropriateness of physical sexual expressions of residents. Physical sexual interactions that are questioned range from sexualized touching or kissing to sexual intercourse. These inquiries often involve questions about whether the activities fall within the scope of sexual abuse.

It is imperative to base a determination of capacity to consent to sexual interactions on a multifaceted assessment of the individual, including consideration of his or her values and interpersonal relationships. A diagnosis of dementia is not an automatic disqualifier for capacity to consent, even though it affects one's ability to communicate. Similarly, a diagnosis of dementia does not routinely entitle family members or anyone else to decide whether a legally competent adult can consent to sexual interactions. On the other hand, people who are cognitively impaired to any extent may need to be protected from sexual abuse. In questionable situations, nurses can initiate interprofessional efforts to assess the older adult's capacity to consent, using guidelines such as those delineated in Box 16.3. In addition to nursing staff, interprofessional team members for this type of assessment may include mental health and medical professionals and professionals from appropriate local agencies such as the Long-Term Care Ombudsman or adult protective services.

BOX 16.3 Guide for Assessing an Older Adult's Capacity to Consent to Physical Sexual Interactions

Does the person understand *all* the following:
- That the act is sexual in nature?
- That one's body is private?
- That he or she has the right to say "no" to any unwanted sexual actions?
- That engagement in certain sexual acts may involve health risks?

Does the person have the ability to express choices about relationships?

Are the sexual interactions enjoyable, pleasurable, or positive in other ways?

Are there indicators of negative effects of the relationship?

Are there indicators of negative consequences of the sexual interactions?

Has the person expressed regret after previously engaging in similar sexual interactions?

Is the relationship consistent with the person's values and personal history?

NURSING RESPONSIBILITIES AND CASE EXAMPLES

The primary nursing responsibility in all situations of suspected physical sexual abuse is to make an immediate report and facilitate a referral for a complete physical examination by a qualified sexual assault professional. In addition, nurses address immediate physical needs and provide appropriate emotional support. If the situation involves prior (rather than current) episodes of suspected abuse or does not involve physical sexual abuse, nurses are responsible for reporting to appropriate agencies, but an immediate physical examination may not be necessary. In all situations of suspected or actual abuse, nurses address the needs of the older adult through direct nursing interventions or by facilitating referrals for appropriate interventions. For example, an appropriate intervention in ongoing situations would be to take actions to protect the victim from unsupervised contact with the alleged offender. Depending on the circumstances, nurses can consider referrals to resources discussed in the section on Resources for Addressing Sexual Abuse of Older Adults, as well as those described in Chapters 10 and 11 (e.g., emergency housing).

In community settings, domestic violence and sexual assault programs may be an important resource for some situations, particularly those involving older adults who are not cognitively impaired. Because these programs are typically based on a self-help model, nurses can encourage victims to call for help. Another strategy is to obtain permission from the victim and directly facilitate a referral by calling the domestic violence program while the person is in the room and involving the person in the phone conversation.

Each of the four cases presented in this section describes a situation of actual sexual abuse that requires nursing interventions. In contrast to the fictitious cases presented in other chapters, these cases were cited in studies based on reviews of adult protective service agency records. Although these cases may seem extreme—and even repulsive—elder abuse scholars have documented many cases that are even more serious. Following each case presentation is a section on nursing responsibilities, which was developed for this chapter and not part of the original case citation.

CASE 16.1   Visiting Nurse Reports Incestuous Sexual Abuse

Mrs. J. is 86 years old and moved into the home of her daughter and son-in-law to recover from a broken hip. Several months later, her daughter died and her son-in-law, Charlie, became her caregiver. Mrs. J. disclosed to her visiting nurse that Charlie took nude photos of her. He undressed her, pulled back all bed clothing, and instructed Mrs. J. to open her legs and smile for the camera. He told her that he needed the photos "so that no one will think I abused you," and said that her daughter would want her to cooperate. Mrs. J. also reported that Charlie had "checked" her genitals by pushing something large in and out of her vagina. While he did this, he told her that she needed to help him climax. In addition, Charlie had forced her to sign papers without the opportunity to determine the content. The nurse filed an elder abuse report triggering criminal and adult protective services investigations, as well as an arrest of Charlie and intervention services

(continued)

CASE 16.1 Visiting Nurse Reports Incestuous Sexual Abuse *(continued)*

for Mrs. J. It was learned that Charlie earned his living as a home health aide (Ramsey-Klawsnik, 2004. Adapted with permission of The Haworth Maltreatment & Trauma Press via Copyright Clearance Center. [Taylor & Francis Ltd, http://www.tandfonline.com/].).

Reflections on Nursing Responsibilities

In this situation, the nurse built upon a trusting relationship and empowered Mrs. J. to disclose details of sexual abuse perpetrated by her son-in-law. The nurse used skillful communication to elicit details and presumably also provided emotional support to Mrs. J. Because of interventions by the visiting nurse, Mrs. J. was protected from further abuse and received ongoing professional services to address her needs.

CASE 16.2 Visiting Nurse Facilitates Appropriate Referrals

Mrs. E. is 80 years old, has Parkinson's disease, and uses a wheelchair. She weighs 95 lbs. and is quite frail. She told her visiting nurse that she was worried about her husband because he exhibited dramatic behavioral changes. These included accusing her of trying to poison him and forcing her into unwanted sexual intercourse. Mr. E. also refused to allow their adult daughter to visit, accusing her of stealing from him and trying to poison him. Mrs. E. reported that until recently her husband had been consistently loving and considerate, not abusive or suspicious. She believed that illness caused the strange behavior. He also experienced short-term memory problems and refused medical help. Mrs. E. did not exhibit the signs and symptoms typically seen in domestic violence victims (such as low self-esteem). Her prime concern was securing treatment for her husband; she had no interest in leaving him or filing criminal charges. The visiting nurse facilitated social services interventions from adult protective services and Mr. E. was involuntarily hospitalized for an evaluation. He was diagnosed with progressive dementia and several other major medical

(continued)

CASE 16.2 Visiting Nurse Facilitates Appropriate Referrals *(continued)*

problems (Ramsey-Klawsnik, 2004. Adapted with permission of The Haworth Treatment & Trauma Press via Copyright Clearance Center. [Taylor & Francis Ltd, http://www.tandfonline.com/].).

Reflections on Nursing Responsibilities

In this situation, the nurse addressed her client's concerns and also identified indicators of sexual and psychological abuse perpetrated by Mrs. E.'s husband. Based on an astute assessment of her client's overall situation, the nurse facilitated social service interventions to assure that Mrs. E. was protected from further abuse. In addition, the nurse supported Mrs. E.'s goal of resolving the abusive situation by addressing her husband's abnormal behaviors. Because of the visiting nurse's interventions, Mr. E. was diagnosed and presumably a plan was initiated to address the needs of both Mr. and Mrs. E.

CASE 16.3 Sexual Abuse in a Nursing Home, Perpetrated by Son

Eighty-three-year-old Mrs. M. resided in a dementia unit of a nursing home, due to prior profound neglect by her son. She had been found sitting naked in a pool of urine, and also wandered her neighborhood alone in a state of undress. Mrs. M. asked nursing home staff when her son would visit, saying that she has sex with him. This statement was attributed to dementia, until a nurse aide witnessed the son placing his hand under Mrs. M's nightgown and touching her genitals while she was seated in a wheelchair. Mrs. M. moved her son's hand away, saying, "No." He then showed her a carton of chocolate milk and said, "Now be a good girl so you can have your chocolate milk." The aide did not immediately report the episode, but instead tried to convince herself that there must be some other explanation for what she saw. Three days later, she described her observation to her supervisor, stating that her conscience required that she report it, since she was certain that she had observed sexual molestation. The nurse did not immediately report the incident to adult protective services or to law enforcement. However, when Mrs. M.'s

(continued)

CASE 16.3 Sexual Abuse in a Nursing Home, Perpetrated by Son *(continued)*

chart was reviewed by a state worker, this incident was discovered along with two additional entries documenting sexual abuse by the son. The facility and supervising nurse faced sanctions by licensing agents; adult protective services obtained a court order to prohibit the son's unsupervised access to Mrs. M. (Ramsey-Klawsnik, 2004, pp. 49–50. Apapted with permission of The Haworth Treatment & Trauma Press via Copyright Clearance Center. [Taylor & Francis Ltd, http://www.tandfonline.com/].).

Reflections on Nursing Responsibilities

Mrs. M.'s situation illustrates one of the many cases of sexual abuse that are overlooked and unreported due to factors such as those discussed in this chapter. This case occurred between 1993 and 2002; perhaps nurses today would recognize it and take action because of their increased awareness about elder abuse. The following interventions have been recommended for addressing alleged sexual abuse of residents of long-term care facilities: (a) Take immediate action when residents report assault, (b) obtain immediate medical care for the alleged victims, (c) leave all evidence intact, (d) document detailed information, (e) notify authorities. On an institutional level, facilities need to have protocols in place for best response and collaborate with adult protective services and law enforcement (Ramsey-Klawsnik & Teaster, 2012).

CASE 16.4 Resident-to-Resident Sexual Abuse in a Nursing Home

Sixty-seven-year-old Mr. N. suffered from chronic mental illness, long-term alcoholism, and a host of physical problems. He required constant supervision and medical management and was placed in a nursing home. Facility staff soon realized that Mr. N. presented a severe supervision challenge in that he was repeatedly found sexually molesting women who resided in the facility. All of his victims were more physically and cognitively impaired than he. Some suffered from

(continued)

CASE 16.4 Resident-to-Resident Sexual Abuse in a Nursing Home (*continued*)

advanced dementia, some were aphasic or paralyzed. Many were assaulted in their beds or wheelchairs. Numerous episodes of sexually offensive behavior toward other residents were charted. None of the psychotropic medications prescribed by Mr. N.'s physicians and psychiatric nurse practitioner were effective and he continued to reside in the facility for more than 6 months, during which time he sexually assaulted many female residents. Family members and guardians of several residents brought suit against the facility, the physicians, and the nurse practitioner for failing to effectively control Mr. N.'s abusive and dangerous behavior. (Ramsey-Klawsnik et al., 2007).

Reflections on Nursing Responsibilities

This situation may seem extreme; however, similar episodes of resident-to-resident sexual abuse can occur in all types of long-term care facilities, including nursing homes, assisted living facilities, and residential care facilities. Although Mr. N.'s physicians and psychiatric nurse practitioner initiated treatments to manage his abusive behaviors, sexual assaults of female residents continued to occur. The pharmacological interventions for Mr. N. were inadequate and other residents were not protected from his abusive behaviors. Nonpharmacological interventions for hypersexual behaviors cited in nursing literature include redirecting behavior, educating and counseling patients, using same-sex caregivers, and using clothing that fastens in the back (Wallace & Safer, 2009).

In addition to direct interventions to address Mr. N.'s behaviors, staff should address the broader context. This situation required reports to appropriate agencies, and all residents involved required services from professionals skilled in addressing sexual assault episodes. For example, adult protective services and the Long-Term Care Ombudsman programs may have provided consultation by professionals who are specially trained to address sexual abuse. Also, a nurse member of the Sexual Assault Nurse Examiners (SANE) program may have provided training or consultation to help staff address this situation. In addition to making reports, nurses need to facilitate the provision of services for older adults who are sexually assaulted.

RESOURCES FOR ADDRESSING SEXUAL ABUSE OF OLDER ADULTS

Although still relatively scarce, specialized resources related to sexual abuse of older adults are developing gradually and several excellent national resources are currently available. The National Sexual Violence Resource Center (NSVRC) opened in 2000 as a national information and resource hub relating to all aspects of sexual violence. Since 2010, the NSVRC has received funds from the Department of Justice, Office on Violence Against Women, to address sexual abuse of older adults. Of particular relevance to nurses is an online information packet with information about research, resources, and a guide for health care providers.

Community-based resources usually focus on sexual abuse as an aspect of domestic violence, but there is increasing awareness of the need to address these situations as a form of elder abuse. For example, organizations that address domestic violence are working together with adult protective services agencies and other aging network programs to develop coalitions that address the unique needs of sexually abused older adults. In 1999, the Wisconsin Coalition Against Domestic Violence developed the National Clearinghouse on Abuse in Later Life (NCALL) as a resource and training center to help communities develop a coordinated response to domestic and sexual abuse in later life. The resources listed at the end of this section provide up-to-date information about national and local programs that are helpful for addressing abuse in later life.

Faith-based organizations are also developing programs to address issues related to domestic violence and elder abuse. In 2008, NCALL and Safe Havens Interfaith Partnership Against Domestic Violence have worked together to provide technical assistance to programs that receive grants from the Department of Justice, Office on Violence Against Women. Older women who are experiencing or have experienced domestic sexual abuse may benefit from participation in support groups and other local resources available through domestic violence programs.

Older women participating in support groups for elder sexual abuse

- "I thought I was the only one living like this."
- "When I hear the stories, I think we were all married to the same man."
- "I always thought it would get better."
- "I tried not to think about the abuse. He told me he was just keepin' me in line, that I'd best not get uppity about it."
- "I just learned to work around it. What else could I do? I loved him, for the most part, and divorce was too scandalous to consider. I was a good wife."

(Wisconsin Coalition Against Domestic Violence, 2010).

Nurses working in acute care settings usually have access to specialized resources, such as those provided through SANE. In 2016, more than 700 SANE professionals are available throughout the United States to provide direct and specialized services to address the complex needs of victims of sexual assault. The SANE program focuses primarily on care for victims of physical sexual assault; however, a SANE professional may be able to provide staff education in long-term facilities or community-based organizations to help staff identify and address sexual abuse of older adults, as in Case 16.4.

When sexual abuse occurs in long-term care facilities, the nursing home ombudsman program can help address consequences for all involved, including the needs of the older adult in the broader context, as discussed in Chapter 4. They may also be able to provide staff education about the prevention of and interventions for sexual abuse, particularly with regard to resident-to-resident abuse and when issues related to residents' rights are involved.

Contact Information for Resources Related to Sexual Abuse of Older Adults

- Interfaith Partnership Against Domestic Violence, www .interfaithpartners.org
- NCALL, www.ncall.us
- National Domestic Violence Hotline, available 24/7, 800-799-7233 or www.ndvh.org
- National Sexual Violence Resource Center, www.nsvrc.org
- SANE, www.forensicnurses.org

KEY POINTS: WHAT NURSES NEED TO KNOW AND CAN DO

- Despite the myths and misconceptions surrounding sexual abuse of older adults, accurate information about this topic is increasingly more available (Table 16.1, Box 16.1).
- Nurses need to be keenly aware of their serious responsibility to observe for indicators of sexual abuse, particularly in older adults who have dementia, and to assess the situation when indicators are identified (Box 16.2).
- A comprehensive assessment of an older adult's capacity to consent to sexual interactions is required in many situations,

particularly when one or more of the involved individuals are cognitively impaired (Box 16.3).

- Nurses cannot reverse the effects of sexual abuse that has already occurred, but they can prevent further abuse by recognizing indicators, making reports, and facilitating referrals for appropriate intervention (Cases 16.1–16.4).

REFERENCES

Burgess, A. W. (2006). *Elderly victims of sexual abuse and their offenders.* Washington, DC: U.S. Department of Justice. Retrieved from www.ncjrs.gov/pdffiles1/nij/grants/216550.pdf

Burgess, A., Ramsey-Klawsnik, H., & Gregorian, S. (2008). Comparing routes of reporting in elder sexual abuse cases. *Journal of Elder Abuse & Neglect, 20,* 336–352.

National Center on Elder Abuse. (2007). *Major types of elder abuse.* Retrieved from www.ncea.aoa.gov

Ramsey-Klawsnik, H. (2004). Elder abuse within the family. *Journal of Elder Abuse & Neglect, 15,* 43–58.

Ramsey-Klawsnik, H. (2012). *Research to practice brief: The study of sexual abuse of vulnerable adults in care facilities.* National Adult Protective Services Resource Center. Retrieved from www.napsanow.org

Ramsey-Klawsnik, H., & Teaster, P. B. (2012). Sexual abuse happens in healthcare facilities—What can be done to prevent it? *Generations, 36*(3), 53–59.

Ramsey-Klawsnik, H., Teaster, P. B., Mendiondo, M. S., Abner, E. L., Cecil, K. A., & Tooms, M. R. (2007). Sexual abuse of vulnerable adults in care facilities: Clinical findings and a research initiative. *Journal of the American Psychiatric Nurses Association, 12,* 332–339.

Ramsey-Klawsnik, H., Teaster, P. B., Mendiondo, M. S., Marcum, J. L., & Abner, E. L. (2008). Sexual predators who target elders: Findings from the first national study of sexual abuse in care facilities. *Journal of Elder Abuse & Neglect, 20,* 353–376.

Teaster, P. B., Ramsey-Klawsnik, H., Mendiondo M. S., Abner, E., Cecil, K., & Tooms, M. (2007). From behind the shadows: A profile of the sexual abuse of older men residing in nursing homes. *Journal of Elder Abuse & Neglect, 19,* 29–45.

Wallace, M., & Safer, M. (2009). Hypersexuality among cognitively impaired older adults. *Geriatric Nursing, 30,* 230–237.

Wiglesworth, A., & Mosqueda, L. (2011). *People with dementia as witnesses to emotional events.* U.S. Department of Justice. Retrieved from www.ncjrs.gov/pdffiles1/nij/grants/234132.pdf

Wisconsin Coalition Against Domestic Violence. (October 2010). Advocacy for survivors of abuse in later life. *Coalition Chronicles, 29*(2). Available at www.wcadv.org.

EPILOGUE

Georgia J. Anetzberger

The past decade has witnessed unprecedented interest and activity around elder abuse. There were more scholarly articles in a wider array of journals, more news accounts of specific incidents, and more multidisciplinary networking nationwide than ever before. Also, new champions emerged, joining pioneers and stalwarts, to create greater public awareness, professional understanding, and tested practices for responding to elder abuse. Throughout, nurses, including those in clinical settings, have been visible and involved.

Moreover, within the health care system, an evolution is underway, moving the perception of and approach to elder abuse from simply that of a medical syndrome to also that of a public health issue. This underscores growing recognition that only addressing elder abuse once it has occurred is costly in terms of suffering and interventions. In contrast, preventing elder abuse from happening in the first place is more humane and likely to be less expensive.

Although both approaches had their origins in the 1970s, elder abuse as a medical syndrome has dominated since, in part by medicine aligning itself with criminal justice during recent decades when societal trends emphasized the medicalization of more and more maladies and the criminalization of more and more unacceptable behaviors. The end result was collaboration on such elder abuse–related initiatives as establishing forensic markers and conducting fatality reviews.

Elder abuse as a public health issue came into its own more slowly. Although U.S. Surgeon General Louis Sullivan included elder abuse in his 1989 Task Force on Family Violence, real public health interest was delayed until the past several years. Its eventual emergence is evidenced in forums like the 2013 Workshop on Elder Abuse and Its Prevention, sponsored by the Institute of Medicine, and the 2015 Multiple Approaches to Understanding and Preventing Elder Abuse and Mistreatment Workshop, sponsored by the National Institute of Health. It is noteworthy that each forum has included nurses in leadership and participant roles, their contributions illustrated in specific recommendation content and targeted practice settings. Generally, such forums result in a set of recommendations for moving the field forward. Unfortunately, after galvanizing attention on elder abuse and enthusiasm to address it, forums are too frequently forgotten and their recommendations are never implemented.

A contrast is found in the Elder Justice Roadmap, perhaps the most important set of elder abuse–related recommendations developed to date. Released in August 2014, the Roadmap represents a strategic plan resource "by the field, for the field" (Connolly, Brandl, & Breckman, 2014, p. 2). Funded by the U.S. Department of Justice with support from the U.S. Department of Health and Human Services, it is a 122-page document that examines elder abuse, its human and economic toll, and response challenges before listing 121 action recommendations across the four domains of direct service, education, policy, and research. Together, these identified priorities suggest what needs to be accomplished and offers every person, discipline, organization, community, and government level a potential role to "commit to combat" elder abuse, in the words of Assistant Secretary of Aging Kathy Greenlee.

Compared with previous efforts, the Roadmap involved more stakeholders in identifying critical priorities and used more diverse methods for gathering input, including concept mapping, facilitated discussions, leadership interviews, and dialogue summits. Uniquely, it also put in place structures to help facilitate recommendation implementation. These include a steering committee and e-mail address for reporting experience and progress. In addition, the current iteration of the National Center on Elder Abuse established a task agenda that focuses on implementing selected Roadmap recommendations.

Nursing, and especially clinical nursing, is reflected throughout the Roadmap recommendations. For nurses, relevant recommendations from the domain of direct services include developing measures to protect those receiving long-term services and supports, to enlarge the formal caregiver workforce and ensure adequate compensation and working conditions, and to understand the imperative of cultural capacity in responding to elder abuse. With respect to the domain of education, relevant recommendations include creating a national elder abuse education and training strategic plan and assuring that long-term care providers are trained in person-centered care. In the domain of policy, recommendations relevant to nursing include strengthening the monitoring of long-term services and supports and establishing policy to respond to transitions that might heighten elder abuse risk. Finally, for the domain of research, relevant recommendations include undertaking studies that determine the effectiveness of elder abuse interventions, develop better instruments to assess whether potential victims have cognitive impairments, and delineate the characteristics of elder abuse victims and perpetrators.

Implementation of the previously cited Roadmap recommendations relevant to nursing would not only facilitate improved clinical practice for the discipline, it is also critical to "combating" elder abuse as a health problem overall. Collectively, successful recommendation implementation would mean that practitioners are educated and trained on elder abuse and related interventions, and able to identify, report, and respond to abuse occurrence across settings quickly and effectively. It would mean that cognitive impairment can be thoroughly assessed and appropriately used in care planning and service provision. It would mean that practitioners work in settings that support abuse prevention and intervention and assure that practitioners function under conditions that promote professional competency, cultural capacity, and personal wellness. It would mean that interdisciplinary and intersystem activity around elder abuse was routine and embraced, sanctioned in public policy and well-funded. It would mean that existing elder abuse interventions are evidence-based and sufficiently available to impact the problem wherever it occurs. Finally, and perhaps most importantly, it would mean that enough understanding of elder abuse exists around its risk factors and applicable community resources that meaningful elder abuse prevention is possible and promoted in every locale.

This seemingly utopian image for elder abuse understanding and response is not impossible, and clinical nurses can play meaningful roles in making it a reality. It almost goes without saying that clinical nurses make invaluable contributions to the domain of direct service, providing assessments and care, teaching and coaching, advocacy and support for individual patients and their families in multiple settings and situations. Assuming this role, however, also enables clinical nurses to impact the remaining domains of education, policy, and research. By way of illustration, for education, clinical nurses can identify training gaps and facilitate the learning of service providers under their direction. For policy, clinical nurses can make known regulatory issues that deserve attention and provide case studies for legislative testimony. Finally, for research, clinical nurses can suggest priorities for investigation, provide data, and give meaning to study results.

Bottom line, the field of elder abuse is best served when clinical nurses go beyond their traditional role in direct service and make contributions to the other domains as well. The former fosters betterment on an individual basis, the latter for systems and society overall. Both are critical to advancing elder abuse understanding and response, and both are suitable arenas for clinical nurses. Guidance for action is found in the Elder Justice Roadmap. Clinical nurses are charged with becoming familiar with the document and its implications. The concluding statement in the Roadmap leaves little doubt with respect to "next steps." "There is a role for everyone. The time to act is now" (Connolly et al., 2014, p. 32).

REFERENCE

Connolly, M.-T., Brandl, B., & Breckman, R. (2014). The Elder Justice Roadmap: A stakeholder initiative to respond to an emerging health, justice, financial and social crisis. Washington, DC: U.S. Department of Justice and U.S. Department of Health and Human Services.

EPILOGUE

Terry Fulmer

There are more than 3 million nurses in the United States. According to the World Health Organization, more than 85% of all care delivered globally is done so by the nursing profession. Imagine if we could capture the power of our nursing workforce and bring that talent to bear upon the serious syndrome of elder mistreatment. I use the term *elder mistreatment* because I think of it as the outcome of the serious adverse events that follow abuse, neglect, exploitation, and abandonment. In any form, detecting actions that create a state of elder mistreatment can and must be a part of our nursing assessment and care planning for the well-being of older adults in every setting. This book describes the possibilities and reminds us that every touch point with our patients, our clients, our residents, regardless of setting, is a moment to ask if elder mistreatment is present and what we will do about it. A major stumbling block has always been the fear of finding a case and not knowing what to do next. This important book guides nurses in their practice as they consider the different types of elder mistreatment and what their respective actions can and should be.

When nurses see patients in a crisis state, as in emergency departments, the immediate nursing practice is to screen and intervene, as there is a fear for the patients' safety. This may include a protective service call or protective admission to the hospital until a safe haven can be found. This is an unpopular step given the complexities of payment mechanisms and concern regarding the necessary restriction of the older person. The astute nurses will know to bring their administrators and team members into the assessment and care planning for optimal results.

For nurses with an ongoing relationship with an older person, changes in cognition should be an immediate warning sign. As noted in this book, it is well documented that cognitive impairment is a risk factor for elder mistreatment. Cognitive impairment puts the older person in a vulnerable state where not only is there a lack of capacity to tell a meaningful story about what is going on, but even more importantly, cognitive impairment creates doubt on the side of clinicians regarding the veracity of the subjective history given by the older adult. In this moment, nurses know that the older person is extremely vulnerable and even more vigilance is required to ensure his or her safety.

Nurses know how to treat family systems and understand that none of us lives in a vacuum. The elder caregiver dyad is a complex system and may include two or more people who have long-standing histories together that are always delicate and challenging to fully comprehend. If the older person had been abusive to his or her child, and the child is now the adult caregiver, any of us can imagine that the relationship will be uneven at best and care planning will be complex. The ability to recognize this complexity and invite social workers, psychiatrists, and clinical psychologists into the care planning is a particular strength of nursing practice. It has been said that nurses are the caregivers and integrators on the health care team. We are the clinical discipline available 24 hours a day, seven days a week, and are frequently the hub of the narrative that surrounds the older adult. Nurses need to ensure that they are facile with documentation in electronic health records that can be readily understood by the care team in complex cases of elder mistreatment. Books like this are essential for all of us in our knowledge building as we address cases of elder mistreatment. I am indebted to the Beth Israel Hospital Elder Abuse Team in Boston, MA, for my early formation as an expert nurse in this field and wish to express my gratitude to Dr. Joyce Clifford, Dr. Mitchell T. Rabkin, Dr. Trish Gibbons, and Mrs. Sandi Fenwick for their support for improving clinical excellence in elder mistreatment practice.

Further, I present my deepest respect and admiration to all the nurses who work tirelessly to improve the quality of life for older adults everywhere.

APPENDIX A: CONTACT INFORMATION FOR STATE ADULT PROTECTIVE SERVICE AGENCIES FOR REPORTING ELDER ABUSE

Contact information for some states is listed on website according to county.

Check websites for online reporting forms.

Alabama (334) 242-1350
http://dhr.alabama.gov/directory/Adult_Prot_Svcs.aspx

Alaska (907) 269-3666
http://dhss.alaska.gov/dsds/Pages/aps/default.aspx

Arizona (877) 767-2385
https://des.az.gov/services/aging-and-adult/independent-living/long-term-care-ombudsman

Arkansas, Division of Aging and Adult Services
(800) 482-8049, http://www.daas.ar.gov/

California (by county)
http://www/cdss.ca.gov/agedblinddisabled/PG1298.htm

Colorado (by county)
http://www.coloradoaps.com

Connecticut (in state) 1-888-385-4225, (out of state) 1-800-203-1234
http://www.ct.gov/dss/cwp/view.asp?A=2353&Q-305232

Delaware (800) 223-9074
http://dhss.delaware.gov/dsaapd/aps.html

District of Columbia (202) 541-3950
http://dhs.dc.gov/service/adult-protective-services

Florida (800) 962-2873
https://reportabuse.dcf.state.fl.us

Georgia (800) 866-552-4464
http://aging.dhs.georgia.gov/adult-protective-services?vgnextoid=
018267b27edb0010Vgn

Hawaii (808) 832-5115
http://humanservices.hawaii.gov/ssd/home/adult-services

Idaho (208) 334-3833
http://aging.idaho.gov/protection

Illinois (866) 800-1409
http://www.illinois.gov/aging/Pages/default.aspx

Indiana (800) 992-6978
http://www.in.gov/fssa/da/3479.htm

Iowa (800) 362-2178
http://dhs.iowa.gov/dependent_adult_abuse

Kansas (800) 922-5330
http://www.dcf.ks.gov/services/PPS/Pages.KIPS/KIPS/
WebIntake.aspx

Kentucky (877) 597-2331
http://www.chfs.ky.gov/dcbs/dpp/Adult+Protective+and+General+
Adult+Services.htm

Louisiana (800) 898-4910
http://www.dhh.louisiana.gov/index.cfm/page/120/n/126

Maine (800) 624-8404
http://www.maine.gov/dhhs/oads/aps-guardianship/
index.html

Maryland (800) 917-7383
http://www.dhr.state.md.us/blog/?page_id=4531

Massachusetts (800) 922-2275
http://www.mass.gov/elders/service-orgs-advocates/protective-
services-program.html

Michigan (855) 444-3911
www.michigan.gov/mdhhs

Minnesota (844) 880-1574
http://www.mn.gov/dhs/reportadultabuse

Mississippi (800) 222-8000
http://www.mdhs.state.ms.us/programs-and-services-for-seniors/
adult-protective-services

Missouri (800) 392-0210
http://health.mo.gov/safety/abuse

Montana (800) 551-3191
http://dphhs.mt.gov/SLTC/APA.aspx

Nebraska (800) 652-1999
http://dhhs.ne.gov/children_family_services/Pages/nea_aps_aps
index.aspx

Nevada (888) 729-0571
http://adsd.nv.gov/Programs/Seniors/EPS/EPS_Prog

New Hampshire (800) 949-0470 or (603) 271-7014
http://www.dhhs.nh.gov/dcbcs/beas/adultprotection.htm

New Jersey (800) 792-8820
http://www.state.nj.us/humanservices/doas/service/aps

New Mexico (866) 654-3219 or (505) 476-4912
http://www.nmaging.state.nm.us/Adult_ProtectiveServices.aspx

New York (844) 697-3505
http://ocfs.ny.gov/main/psa

North Carolina (by county)
http://www.ncdhhs.gov/assistance/adult-services/adult-protective-services

North Dakota (855) 462-5465
http://www.nd.gov/dhs/services/adultsaging/vulnerable.html

Ohio (by county)
http://www.aging.ohio.gov

Oklahoma (405) 521-3660
http://www.okdhs.org/services/aps/pages/default.aspx

Oregon (855) 503-7233
http://www.oregon.gov/DHS/ABUSE/Pages/index.aspx

Pennsylvania (800) 490-8505
http://www.portal.state.pa.us/portal/server.pt/community/abuse_or_crime/17992

Rhode Island (401) 462-0555
http://www.dea.ri.gov/programs/protective_services.php

South Carolina (803) 898-7318
http://aging.sc.gov/Pages/default.aspx

South Dakota (605) 773-3656
https://dss.sd.gov/asa/services/adultprotective.aspx

Tennessee (888) 277-8366
http://www.tennessee.gov/humanservices/article/adult-protective-services

Texas (800) 252-5400
http://www.dfps.state.tx.us/Adult_Protection

Utah (800) 371-7897
http://daas.utah.gov/adult-protective-services

Vermont (802) 871-3326 or in Vermont only (800) 564-1612
http://www.dlp.vermont.gov/protection/abuse-reproting-form

Virginia (888) 832-3858
http://www.dss.virginia.gov/family/as/aps.cgi

Washington (by county)
https://www.dshs.wa.gov/altsa/home-and-community-services/
reporting-abuse

West Virginia (800) 352-6513
http://www.dhhr.wv.gov/bcf/Pages/default.aspx

Wisconsin (by county)
https://www.dhs.wisconsin.gov/long-term-care-support/elderly-
services/elder-abuse

Wyoming (307) 777-3602
https://sites.google.com/a/wyo.gov/dfsweb/social-services/adult-
protective-services-aps

APPENDIX B: CONTACT INFORMATION FOR STATE LONG-TERM CARE OMBUDSMAN PROGRAMS

Alabama, Long-Term Care Ombudsman
(800) 243-9596, http://adss.alablama.gov/long-term-care.html

Alaska, Mental Health Trust Authority, Office of the State LTC Ombudsman
(907) 334-4483, http://www.akoltco.org

Arizona, Division of Aging and Adult Services
(602) 542-6615, https://des.az.gov/services/aging-and-adult/independent-living/long-term-care-ombudsman

Arkansas, Division of Aging and Adult Services
(501) 682-8952, http://www.arombudsman.com

California, Department of Aging
(916) 419-7510, http://www.aging.ca.gov/programs/#LTCOP

Colorado, The Legal Center
(800) 288-1376 x510 http://www.colorado.gov/cs/Satellite/CDHS-VetDis/CBON/1251595460161

Connecticut, State Department on Aging
(860) 424-5200, http://www.ltcop.state.ct.us

Delaware, State LTC Ombudsman
(302) 255-9390, http://dhss.delaware.gov/dsaapd/ltcop.html

District of Columbia, Long-Term Care Ombudsman Office, Legal
Counsel for the Elderly
(202) 434-2140 or (202) 434-2190, http://www.aarp.org/states/dc/LCE

Florida, State LTC Ombudsman
(850) 414-2331, http://ombudsman.myflorida.com

Georgia, Office of the State LTC Ombudsman, Division of Aging
Services, Department of Human Services
(404) 657-5327 or (404) 416-0211, http://www.georgiaombudsman.org

Hawaii, Executive Office on Aging
(808) 586-0100, http://hawaii.gov/health/eoa/LTCO.html

Idaho, Commission on Aging
(208) 334-3833, http://www.idahoaging.com/ombudsman/index.html

Illinois, Department on Aging
(217) 785-3143, http://www.illinois.gov/aging/Pages/default.aspx

Indiana, Office of the LTC Ombudsman
(800) 622-4484 or (317) 232-4134, http://www.in.gov/fssa/da/3474
.html

Iowa, Department on Aging
(515) 725-3333, http://iowaaging.gov/long-term-care-ombudsman

Kansas, Office of the State LTC Ombudsman
(785) 296-3017, http://da.state.ks.us/care

Kentucky, Nursing Home Ombudsman Agency of the Bluegrass
(859) 277-9215 or (800) 372-2991, http://www.ombuddy.org

Louisiana, Governor's Office of Elderly Affairs
(225) 342-7100, http://goea.louisiana.gov/index.cfm?md=pagebuild
er&tmp=home&pid=4&pnid=2&nid=15

Maine, LTC Ombudsman Program
(207) 621-1079, http://www.maineombudsman.org

Maryland, Department of Aging
(410) 767-2161, http://www.aging.maryland.gov/Ombudsman.html

Massachusetts, Office of Elder Affairs, State LTC Ombudsman
(617) 727-7750, http://www.mass.gov/elders/service-orgs-advocates/
ltc-ombudsman

Michigan, Office of Services to the Aging, State LTC Ombudsman
(517) 335-0148, http://www.michigan.gov/miseniors

Minnesota, Office of the Ombudsman for Long-Term Care
(651) 431-2553 or (800) 657-3591, http://www.mnaging.net

Mississippi, Division of Aging and Adult Services, Mississippi
Department of Human Services
(601) 359-4927, http://www.mdhs.state.ms.us

Missouri, Division of Senior and Disability Services
(800) 309-3282, http://health.mo.gov/seniors/ombudsman

Montana, Local/Regional Ombudsman Program
(800) 332-2272, http://dphhs.mt.gov/sltc/aging/longtermcareom
budsman.aspx

Nebraska, Division of Medicaid and LTC State Unit on Aging
(402) 471-9345, http://dhhs.ne.gov/medicaid/Aging/Pages/ltcom
bud.aspx

Nevada, Division of Aging and Disability Services
(775) 687-0818, http://www.aging.state.nv.us

New Hampshire, Office of the LTC Ombudsman
(603) 271-4375, http://www.dhhs.nh.gov/oltco/index.htm

New Jersey, Office of Ombudsman for the Institutionalized Elderly
(877) 582-6995, http://www.nj.gov/ooie

New Mexico, Department of Aging and LTC Services
(505) 476-4790, http://www.nmaging.state.nm.us/Long_Term_Om
budsman.aspx

New York, State Office for the Aging
(518) 408-1469 or (518) 473-8718 or 1 (855) 582-6769, http://www.ltc
ombudsman.ny.gov

North Carolina, Division of Aging and Adult Services
(919) 855-3433, http://ncdhhs.gov/assistance/adult-services/long-
term-care-ombudsman

North Dakota, LTC Ombudsman Program, Division of Aging Services
(701) 328-4617, http://www.nd.gov/dhs/services/adultsaging/omb
udsman.html

Ohio, Department of Aging
(800) 282-1206, http://www.aging.ohio.gov

Oklahoma, LTC Ombudsman Program, Division of Aging Services,
Department of Human Services
(405) 521-6734, www.okdhs.org/services/pages/default.aspx

Oregon, State LTC Ombudsman
(800) 522-2602, http://www.oregon.gov/LTCO/Pages/index.aspx

Pennsylvania, Department on Aging
(717) 783-1550, http://www.aging.state.pa.us

Rhode Island, State LTC Ombudsman
(401) 785-3340, http://www.dea.ri.gov/programs/nursing_homes
.php

South Carolina, State LTC Ombudsman, Lt. Governor's Office
on Aging
(803) 734-9900, www.aging.sc.gov/programs/ombudsman/Pages/
default.aspx

South Dakota, Division of Adult Services and Aging, Department of
Social Services
(605) 773-3656, www.dss.sd.gov/asa/services/ombudsman.aspx

Tennessee, State LTC Ombudsman, Tennessee Commission on
Aging and Disability
(615) 253-4392, http://www.tn.gov/aging/topic/long-term-care-
ombudsman

Texas, Department of Aging and Disability Services, Center for Consumer and External Affairs
(800) 252-2412, http://www.dads.state.tx.us/news_info/ombuds man/index.html

Utah, LTC Ombudsman Program, Division of Aging and Adult Services, Department of Human Services
(801) 538-3924, http://www.hsdaas.utah.gov/ombudsman/index .html

Vermont, State LTC Ombudsman, Vermont Legal Aid, Inc.
(802) 863-5620 or 1 (800) 889-2047, http://www.vtlegalaid.org/ vermont-long-term-care-ombudsman

Virginia, Department for Aging and Rehabilitative Services
(804) 726-6624, http://www.elderrightsva.org

Washington, State LTC Ombudsman Program, Multi-Service Center
(800) 562-6028, http://www.waombudsman.org

West Virginia, State LTC Ombudsman, Aging and Disability Resource Center
(304) 363-1595, http://www.wvseniorservices.gov

Wisconsin, Board on Aging and Long Term Care
(800) 815-0015, http://longtermcare.state.wi.us

Wyoming, Office of the State Long-Term Care Ombudsman, Wyoming Senior Citizens, Inc.
(307) 777-8225, http://www.wyomingseniors.com

INDEX

Note: Page numbers followed by *f, t, b,* or *c* represent figures, tables, boxes, or cases respectively.